Table of Contents

Introduction

"Performance is not determined by your conditions but by your actions."

If you're one of many who finds themselves confused and overwhelmed with the deluge of information that surrounds the health and fitness industry, then this book is for you: the person who demands more, the person who isn't satisfied with trending fitness crazes, the person who wants the real story and understands that physical greatness isn't achieved through crash diets and infomercial products, but through sound principals and best practices.

I believe deeply that when given the right information it becomes increasingly difficult to make the wrong decisions. This book is to serve as a road map and compass to keep you focused on your journey to physical prowess, and arm you with the proper defense against false information. We live in a time where companies spend billions to grab your attention with catchy headlines like "Rapid Fat Loss", "Six Weeks to a Six Pack", and so on. That is fantasy, a story they are working tirelessly to get you to believe in hopes that you'll buy their product. The reality is that life does not allow extreme results to happen instantaneously. Anything worth doing takes time, and how we spend our time is one of the few things we have control of.

We must take responsibility for our lives. We can't blame the bread companies, big Pharma, or home workout DVDs for duping us into believing that the answers we seek are in a slice of whole wheat toast, magic pill, or 5-minute home workout. We must model our lives after those who have already achieved that in which we seek, and are winning at the game.

 The Performance Code is your playbook.

In this book we will delve into the mindset of top achievers, compare and contrast various fitness modalities, as well as examine studies done on nutrition, performance, fat loss and strength. We'll break down differing theories on fitness programming, understand what physiological factors are involved in energy production, and learn basic self-care and injury prevention techniques.

When your priority shifts to training movements instead of muscles, and your appearance becomes a consequence of your fitness, then you have become a true athlete. You have joined the elite few whose quest for physical performance is not outweighed by their ego's desire for immediate results. During the ladder's lifetime of fits and starts to no avail, the elite few will have not only reaped the health benefits of sound functional movements and best nutrition practices, but will have also achieved a body worthy of magazine covers.

If you're ready to do the work then consider this your call to action.

- Justin Schollard

Chapter 1
Origins
Primal Beginnings

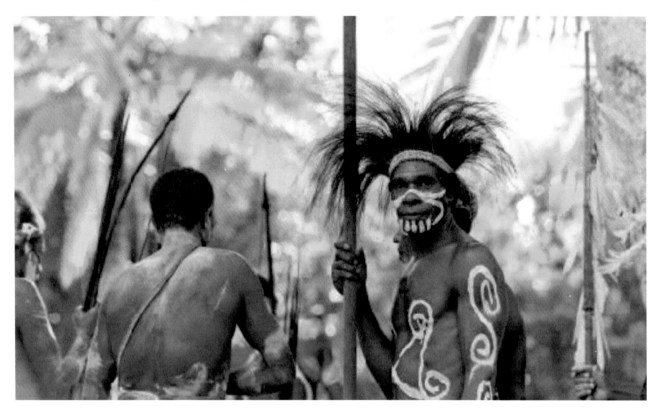

In the beginning, the need for food and shelter was paramount. All of life's daily activities were based around securing one more day of existence. Both the words "hunter" and "gatherer" imply movement as a means of survival. Over the millenniums, our bodies evolved to move dynamically through the world in an amazing variety of patterns and planes. These movement patterns transferred to the ability to wield different external loads like spears, rocks, and animal carcasses. Operating in different modalities, like speed, duration, and repetition, catapulted us to the top of the food chain.

However, without any predatory features like claws or K9 teeth, life was arduous for our early ancestors. Our evolutionary advantage was the ability to run long distances, make tools and weapons, and most importantly, think. It wasn't long before we used our large brains to connect the dots that if sharp objects could puncture skin, imagine what thrusting these objects could do to our prey? So began the development and evolution of rudimentary weapons and techniques to generate force from throwing, thrusting, or swinging an object through space.

It also was not long before we realized that we could be much more efficient hunters by working together in packs. Through years of pattern recognition, we developed the skill of animal tracking; with our unique ability to run long distances, we could literally chase animals down until they collapsed from exhaustion.

In his book, "The Art of Tracking the Origin of Science", Louis Liebenberg asserts that modern science and mathematics can be traced back to early man's tracking ability. Judging the freshness and depth of animal tracks, the time they were left, and speed in which the animal was traveling, allowed our ancestors to extrapolate how far away their potential dinner was, and if it was worth pursuing. This ability created the framework for how we apply calculus and physics to projects today.

Modern sports teams can be linked back to the hunting packs of early man as well; obsession with competition and team sports is hard wired into our psyche. The rush of brain chemicals we get from playing an intense game of football isn't too far from the feeling a pack of hunters, or a band of warriors got when closing in on prey, or battling neighboring tribes.

Thankfully we've evolved passed the primal era of "kill or be killed". However, it's important to understand our heritage and the evolutionary purpose of our vast array of amazing movement abilities. With this understanding we can make smarter choices in order to fully express our genetic potential.

Every type of movement pattern from olympic weightlifting, calisthenics, running, martial arts, plyometric, and strength training spawned from an ancient necessity for survival. Contrary to the relative ease of modern life where food is hardly scarce and the only movement required being to eat and to use the toilet. At the pace we're going, even that could likely be automated in the near future.

Unfortunately, our genetics still resemble that of our hunter gatherer past. Aside from a few short breaks to rest from the heat, a typical day involved moving, foraging, hunting, and exploring until the sun set. Given the contrast of how most of us use our bodies today, it's no wonder we're suffering from massive health epidemics. In fact, for many of us in the developed world, our days are almost the exact opposite of what our bodies were evolved to do; virtually zero movement combined with gross over consumption of processed foods with little nutritional value. What's the number one prescription for avoiding nearly all metabolic disease? Movement.

Our body is perfectly engineered to be a movement machine that works harmoniously with our brain's ability to think strategically and visualize potential outcomes. A first in Earth's history, the psycho-somatic relationship was the corner stone of human survival. Humans could *imagine*. We could hold an image of a finished product in our mind and then use our bodies to manifest it into reality. A total game changer. This branched off into roles and responsibilities within the tribe and every member was expected to contribute to the work that was essential for survival.

This trend continued to evolve (with a few exceptions for royalty and the privileged) right up until the 19th century when mechanization became the craze and all efforts went to inventing new ways to simplify and automate life. The automobile, the sewing machine, super markets and just about anything that could be streamlined, was.

This isn't a bad thing in and of itself. The reason I'm even able to write this book is because of modern technology. Technology has bridged the gap between varying schools of thought, and has allowed teachers and practitioners from all disciplines to create a pool of knowledge that continues to raise the standards from which we all operate.

The other side of that coin is that now entire industries are run exclusively online; plopping it's workforce in front of a computer for 8-12 hours a day. A species that was once not long ago hunting, gathering, running, roaming and foraging is now waking up before the sun, sitting in a chair for breakfast, sitting in their car on the way to work, sitting at their desk, sitting in their car on the way home from work and sitting on the couch until bed. See a problem here?

Until a day returns when sweat equity is the main currency, or when we evolve to a point where we no longer have use for our physical bodies, economics will

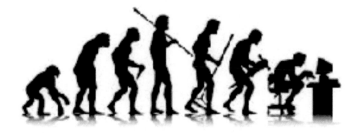

always drive the workplace standards towards maximum productivity. For now, that means sitting your ass in from of a computer much like I am now.

However, this does not doom nor guarantee anything. We absolutely have the ability to express our genetics to their fullest potential and rock a day job simultaneously. We can be both athlete and student, teacher, doctor, plumber, lawyer, cop... whatever. We can stop being a victim of our own evolution and develop a movement practice that will reverse the damage done by years of sedentary lifestyle, improper movement patterns, and poor nutrition. We can become a physical spectacle by harnessing the latest scientific research on functional strength, conditioning and nutrition and applying it to our lives. It's not a secret nor something only a few people with good genetics can achieve. It simply boils down to the choices we make. Deciding between what we want now or what we want most. In other words, discipline.

Our hunter gatherer ancestors didn't really have a choice. They had to be physical or their genes didn't get passed on. They had to chase down prey, climb trees, build shelters and rub sticks together for an extremely long time in order to make fire.

We on the other hand are constantly faced with the decision to take the easy way or the hard way hundreds of times a day. Sadly, most of us choose the easy way. When people ask me how long will it takes to lose 40 lbs. of fat or gain 30 lbs. of muscle, the only answer that makes sense is, "It depends". These goals could take 6 months or a lifetime to be achieved; it really boils down to the day to day choices that keep us in alignment with what we want. Most people don't like to hear this but with 16 years of pattern recognition under my belt, I can honestly tell you that as with anything in life, if it's truly worth doing it's going to take work. So let's get started, shall we?

The Endurance Predator

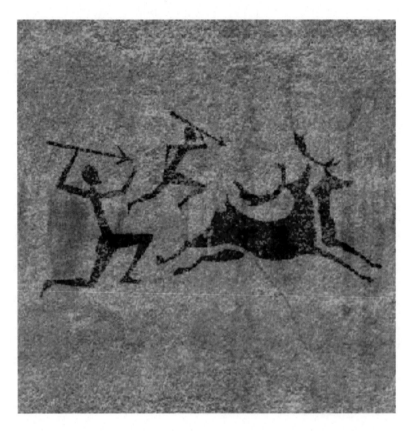

Who are we? How did we last so long without going extinct?

Though many theories exist on the question, the one that makes the most sense to me (other than we just stunk so badly that nothing wanted to eat us.) is that we are a special type of species called an "endurance predator". In his fantastic book, "Born to Run", Christopher McDougall lays out a compelling argument for this. He notes that due to our Achilles tendon, which acts like a spring propelling us forward when running, and our nuchal ligament that connects our scull to our cervical spine (commonly found on animals that run in a head forward position such as horses and dogs) we are in fact born to run.

He notes that unlike other "running species" like quadrupeds (four legged animals) humans have a unique built in cooling system - the ability to sweat and pant while running simultaneously. This might seem like an obvious observation but when you consider that no other animal in the world has this ability it sheds a little light on how our early ancestors hunted. Although quadrupeds are faster off the start than we are, they lack a self-cooling system like sweat, and therefore need to stop and pant about every 400-800 meters. Humans on the other hand, can be trained to literally run for 100 miles straight. No shit. In fact, there are still hunter gatherer tribes existing today in Africa that use endurance as their deadliest weapon. To me it answers the question why anyone in their right mind would want to run a 26-mile marathon or a 100-mile ultra-marathon for that matter. It's just in our DNA. We can out run just about anything until it drops of exhaustion, and becomes easy prey.

This window into our ancient ancestors' hunting practices and our evolution as a species reveals some deeper insight as to why our bodies assimilate calories much more efficiently immediately after a hard workout. It goes beyond the bro science of, "Because it helps you recover faster". Although true, this function of optimal calorie absorption post exertion dates back to our Paleolithic past when after massive effort to find, unearth, run down, or kill, we were finally able to eat. The body, being the amazing adaptational machine it is, recognizes that it better utilize every last calorie as to not waste any precious food energy. In the rare case that our hunter gatherer ancestors came across a gluttony of food, their bodies would simply store the rest of the unneeded energy in the form of body fat that could be used during leaner times. Fast forward to the present day and it is abundantly clear that we are still wired to store unused energy in the form of body fat. The problem now is that the "leaner times" never come. Yet, we continue to store, eat, stay put, repeat.

Fast and Slow Twitch Muscle Fibers

Muscle tissue is comprised of bundles of muscle fibers called myocytes. Each myocyte contains numerous strands of proteins called myofibrils. These myofibrils grab on to each other and pull together, allowing the muscle to contract. These muscle fibers generally fall into two categories, type one (slow twitch) and type 2 (fast twitch).

These muscle types play a large role in how our bodies respond to training. For example, are you a better sprinter than you are a distance runner? If so, then that might indicate a higher composition of type 2 or fast twitch muscle fibers. This means that your body would respond better to short bursts of explosive training. On the contrary, if you find yourself excelling at endurance sports like long distance running or cycling, then that could indicate a higher ratio of type 1 or slow twitch fibers.

Each fiber type is unique in its ability to contract. Although type 1 and 2 fibers produce around the same amount of contractile force, type 2 fibers contract much more quickly, hence the name "fast twitch". They rely on energy that is already stored in the muscle that tends to diminish quickly and takes about 2 to 3 minutes to replenish. Think a max set of pull-ups, full out sprint, or a heavy set of back squats. All of these movements would mainly require the recruitment of type 2 fibers, and all have a finite limit to the duration in which the muscle can perform. These types of movements are considered "anaerobic", meaning the muscle can function without the need for oxygen as energy when training in this way.

Type 1 fibers on the other hand fire much slower, hence their name "slow twitch", but can keep firing for an indefinite amount of time. This is done by metabolizing oxygen as energy, and therefore is called "aerobic". This system becomes increasingly efficient with training.

We'll dive deeper into specific metabolic/energy pathways in a later chapter.

In general, we have about a 50/50 ration of type 1 and 2 fibers, but genetics play a large role in the exact amount an individual has. For example, olympic sprinters often have around 80% type 2 fibers whereas olympic marathon runners have around 80% type 1.

Regardless of your inherited type 1 and 2 compositions, you can reap the advantage of both with the proper training routine. The question on whether one can actually alter the ratio of muscle types by the type of training they do is still undecided. Studies are being done that suggest you can, but nothing conclusive has been disseminated.

To me, this begs the question: why would humans evolve to have both abilities of marathon like endurance and explosive speed and strength? As endurance predators, we would likely chase after prey until the opportune moment to explode in and go for the kill. Like a runner at the end of a marathon who hits the gas on the last 100 meters to pull ahead of the person next to them. Or a basketball player in the fourth quarter of a championship match on a breakaway drive that ends with a slam dunk to win the game.

Type 1 fibers sustain movement for long stretches of time while type 2's give us that turbo boost to push the redline when the stakes are high. When we consider all the various systems in our body, from energy production, muscle recruitment order, and hormone indoctrination, we can start to understand how life was predicated on movement. Hence "Survival of the Fittest". We are indeed movement machines.

Combine the knowledge and understanding of our evolutionary history with modern science, nutrition, and performance and you're left with a raw blueprint of human potential. We have the potential to express our genetics like our early ancestors could never imagine possible due to their uncertain living conditions, access to food, and lack of science. When we focus our training on core foundational movements and do away with trendy fitness distractions that may sound enticing but lack functional application to any real world scenario, we find ourselves with a movement practice that produces sustainable, predictable, and tacit results. These results have the ability to cross over from one modality to the next and develop your movement practice into a skill set that protects you from common injuries caused by unconscious movement patterns, compensatory muscle recruitment, and perhaps most frustrating, misinformation.

Like nearly everything in life the 80/20 principle applies perfectly. In other words, 20% of your actions generate 80% of your results. For this reason, we should take a minimalist approach to our training. As I write this I'm waiting for a client at the gym. Looking around, the people who appear to be the most athletic and proportionate in their body composition aren't the ones with bands strapped to each limb, performing movements with sub-maximal weighs in each hand. It isn't the guy who's always wearing pants to hide his skinny legs (regardless of the temperature) yet just so happens to be training chest and arms again for the 3rd time this week. No, it's the men and women perfecting the basics: squatting, deadlifting, overhead pressing, jumping, slamming, pulling, pushing and twisting in an endless variety of rep ranges, time frames, distances, weight loads, and arrangements.

These people's appearance becomes a consequence of their fitness because they train movements, not muscles. When you approach fitness from this angle it puts purpose behind your training like wind behind your sails; you approach your training like a singer approaches voice lessons. Through your training you're preparing yourself to move through the physical world, immune to unnecessary injury and imbued with the confidence to expand your horizons and try new things without fear of inability.

To reach this level of physical prowess, one must master the basics. Beginning with a fundamental understanding of:

Deadlifting and Squatting.

At this point its cliché to reference how one could go to any developing country and find people everywhere resting in a squat position. It would be even more of an attempt to state the obvious to say how any child under 5 can be observed playing almost effortlessly in a full squat position... But, I'm going for it anyway.

An involuntary "pfft" comes out of my face whenever I read a blog post or article with a trainer or "fitness expert" advising against exercising your legs in any capacity that involves more than sitting down on a machine and extending your knees, or lying down and curling your heals to your butt. Although I disagree entirely, to be honest, I get it. In fact, I would actually prefer someone not try to coach a person through a deadlift or squat who possesses only a vague understanding of the mechanics involved. It's complicated, but only because of the physical state the average American is in.

Believe it or not, there was a time when these movements were second nature to us. Over the centuries we have drifted from this more physical version of ourselves. However, we shouldn't be quick to write off a basic human movement, such as the squat, because of weak arguments such as, "It'll hurt my back."

It falls short in it's attempt to persuade us that something we have been doing since birth, and fundamental to our anatomy, is somehow suddenly dangerous. What I will say is that for the average adult squatting and deadlifting are now learned skills. Those who choose to practice them reap the benefits of a strong, mobile and reliable body.

When our legs are properly trained through squats, deadlifts, lunges, and the like our brain no longer has to recruit the muscles of our lower back to do the job that weak/stiff legs fail to accomplish.

Why do so many of us suffer from back pain? Is it bad luck or genetics? The reason is simple actually. When we sit on our ass for 8-16 hours a day it has consequences. Think about this. We sit while commuting to and from work, sit at the table, and then move to the couch where we remain until bedtime.

If this doesn't sound familiar then great, you made it out. However, if that scenario sounds all too familiar then action is needed to mitigate the damaging effects of prolonged sitting.

Dr. Kelley Starrett of Mobility WOD wrote in his book, "Standing Up to a Sitting World", that for every 2 hours we spend sitting, our life expectancy reduces by 1 hour. He further explains that sitting for 10 hours undoes 90% of the positive effects from a 60-minute workout. Meaning that 60 minute run you did on the treadmill this morning amounts to a 6-minute jog after a full workday spent on your butt.

It isn't my intention to scare you, or to make you feel like you're doomed. Knowledge is power and awareness is the agent of change. When we have the correct information we can avoid the mistakes that leave so many of us confused and in pain. With just a few adjustments to our daily routine, like standing up and mobilizing for 2 minutes every hour, we can significantly alter the damaging effects sitting causes to not only the athlete, but to the desk jockey as well.

As humans we will never stop picking things up from the floor: a dog, a child, a bag of groceries. You name it and most of us at some point in the day will bend over to grab something. Given this reality, why do so many people shy away from training the squat and deadlift? For one, there's a lot of misinformation out there about weight training, and the last thing anyone needs is a back injury from improper form. However, when done correctly, training the squat and deadlift can fix our butt, our back, and our attitude. It can also keep us out of a nursing home at an old age.

Hinging from the waist is fundamental to human movement. The hips are the apex of the body and therefore provide the biggest opportunity to improve our physicality and reclaim our independence. The deadlift is arguably the most functional and beneficial lift of all because it recruits every muscle in your body. When done consistently, you continue to burn fat and build muscle for days after a single workout. We'll dive deeper into squats, deadlifts, and other functional movements in a later chapter. Before we worry about which training routine will finally get us the results we've been looking for our entire life, we gotta get our head straight.

Chapter 2
Mind. Set. Go.
Cultivating the Warrior Spirit

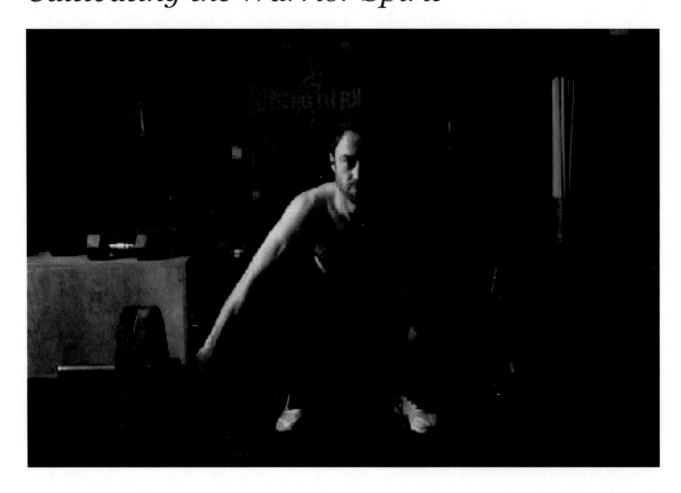

"There is no other road to genius than voluntary self effort"

- Michael Gerber

I've heard all of the excuses, and when strung together it sounds like the same old story that leaves a person with the same old results. Some may be valid: your daughter absolutely needing to get to her music lesson, your wife or husband got sick and left you with all the house choirs, or that email you've been waiting for dropped into your inbox just as you were walking out of the door.

Basically, life happens and will continue to happen. The choice we all have is whether life is happening with us or to us. You may not like to hear that, but it isn't just coincidence that some of the most powerful (and busy) people in the world like Barak Obama, Tony Robins and Steve Aoki prioritize exercise into their daily routine.

I believe that their ability to achieve greatness, and most importantly sustain it, is in large part due to their constant adherence to health and fitness. So, how do we, the average person find time to make health and fitness a priority in our lives? I believe the real question is about energy; what produces it and how do we cultivate it?

First of all, the ego craves status quo, and if left unchecked will continue to make self-limiting, fear based choices that suck the energy right out of us. Until the ego is checked and under control, we will jump from excuse to excuse as to why someone is able to achieve physical, financial or spiritual success but not us, debilitating us from moving forward.

It's the story that we tell ourselves about who we are and what we're capable of that creates the self-limiting belief system which forms the basis of our decision making. Even when we know we need to change, that we hate our current circumstance and want to be better, most of us just won't make a move because no matter how terrible our circumstances may be, it's what we know, and what we know is comfortable. When opportunity presents itself we suddenly catch a bad case of performance paralysis and stand blinking like deer in headlights unable to take a chance.

Change is hard. Trust me I know, but it also happens to be the only constant in life. So, if we're to succeed at anything we must become pros at spotting when it's time to make a move and take action.

We get stuck in our thinking that we can't be more because that would involve doing more, and who has time for that? How am I supposed to carve out an hour a day for exercise when I barely have time to do all the other things in my life? Fair question, and if you can honestly say you spend zero time on social media, binge watching television, or other idle/ low value activities then touché, you got me there. However, we both know that's probably not true.

The American dream has created a culture that idolizes hard work, pulling yourself up by the bootstraps and burning the midnight oil. It's not surprising then that few of us want to admit that we spend on average 20-50% of our day on mindless entertainment. Nobody is saying you shouldn't enjoy a good television episode after a long day. Hell, that's one of the pleasures of life, but that episode, cheat meal, glass of wine or any other indulgence will be ten times more enjoyable when you've taken care of your health and well-being first.

So often I've hid from doing what was necessary in order to become the man I knew I could be. I had no other reason than simply believing the story I was telling myself, that I couldn't pile anything else onto my already busy schedule. Only after taking action did I find that choosing to do more was the very thing that expanded my capacity to be more. This is one of life's paradoxes. This realization came only after I got out of my own way and dropped the self-limiting beliefs that plague so many of us. Good ideas are a dime a dozen, but life meets you at action.

Once we commit to being more, huge obstacles suddenly fall seamlessly into place and clear our path to greatness. It seems counter intuitive, but structure and commitment is what sets us free. Conversely, avoiding structure and commitment keeps us trapped in the throes of life.

When we prepare our meals in advance we no longer waste our time and energy scrambling for food at the last minute. When we create a schedule for ourselves and time block what matters most to us we no longer mindlessly engage in low value activities. This creates the freedom to flourish personally and professionally. Things like exercise become non-negotiable. If you continue to let life happen *to you* then your inner dialogue will always be correct; you don't have time, money, energy, etc. Basically, you cannot be the person you know you should be because you're still doing the same things that keep you the person you are.

As Lau Tzu said "When I let go of who I am, I become what I might be." Spending your day visualizing health, happiness and abundance for all, doesn't mean shit unless you take that first step. Whether you're an athlete or a couch potato the journey to greatness only varies by scale. There is always the next level, the next step and it's up to us to not succumb to complacency and fall into the never ending rat-race where the average person spends a lifetime working 60 hours a week so they can impress coworkers and neighbors with their car, house, wardrobe etc. Even if it means they gain weight rapidly due to lack of sleep, high cortisol levels from stress, too many stimulants and unhealthy foods that just turn into a means of satisfying hunger rather than nourishing their body.

100,000 years ago if you were lucky enough to be born bigger, curvy, stronger or well-endowed you had a good chance of procreating and passing along your genes to the next generation. It was survival of the fittest in its rawest form.

Nowadays things are a little different. It's no longer simply physical prowess that determines your future lineage, its mental. And the part that is physical only applies to our overall state of health and well-being with the slight chance that we'll ever need to use our physicality in a survival situation. So, if it's all about health then why bother achieving the upper echelons of performance? Because of the simple truth that it's always better to have it and not need it, than to need it and not have.

There's arguably no bigger turn off than a macho douchebag picking fights with smaller guys and therefore nothing more satisfying than that smaller guy surprising everyone with his strength and ability to defend himself. Just as with keeping our minds engaged with books, blogs and seminars so too should we adopt a general physical preparedness program to our routine that keep us ready for life's unknowns.

Every single person has a unique genetic potential. We can't all be like Arnold Schwarzenegger but we can express our genes to their highest potential to get us to our personal best. Arnold expressed his, and although not for everyone, body building was his sport and provided him the catalyst to realize his physical potential. It's no different from a swimmer, runner, CrossFitter, or weekend warrior. We all have something that we will be better than average at because all sport has evolved from our innate instinct for competition and from human's unique brand of movement mechanics. As we begin to connect the dots from past to present we see that no matter your physical ambitions adopting a sound strength and conditioning program serves as the foundation to build your goals around. The Performance Code is just that: a catalyst to reaching your unique goals. Whether they be to lose 100 pounds or become a world class athlete, the journey of a thousand miles begins with the first step. Often that first step is getting your head straight and adopting the warrior spirit.

The Warrior Spirit

It should be noted that when I use the word "spiritual" I am not referring to religion, but to the vision we all have of our best self. The vision of the person we know we could be if we committed 100%, got real about who we are and what kind of impact we want to make during our short time on earth. One of my favorite quotes is, "Conquer death and you'll conquer life." I interpret this as, by realizing your own mortality you gain a new respect for time, stopping at nothing to accomplish your dreams. Set yourself free of the bondage society has placed on you since birth and dare to live with purpose. Drop the bullshit excuses and start viewing yourself as an artist with life as your canvas.

In his book, "The Four Agreements", Don Miguel Ruiz explains that,

> "The quest of the spiritual warrior is for personal freedom. Personal Freedom means freedom from fear, illusions, and the fear based beliefs in the mind. In essence, it means to win the war over the beliefs in the mind. It is with Personal Freedom that we are free of the human condition of emotional suffering. Spiritual traditions around the world have their own names for this state of awareness including nirvana and heaven. It is a state that is simply described as living your life with unconditional love, gratitude, and respect, for yourself, and for others."

Everyday we have a choice to be victims or to be warriors. Victims believe that life happens to them, and complain about their circumstances. Warriors participate with and direct their life as it unfolds. Refraining from complaining and casting blame for their circumstances. Warriors take full responsibility for everything they are, because only when you hold yourself accountable can you gain true mastery of self. You're in the driver's seat. If you're out of shape, broke, or no fun to be around the responsibility is on you. When you accept this truth, you become empowered. A "victim mindset" would lead you to believe that the world must change before you are able to make a change. Warriors know this sentiment to be false because the only things in the world we can change are our thoughts and our deeds.

I've been there. Face to face with a pending workout with absolutely zero motivation to start. Buying into my own inner dialogue of, "Maybe I should just rest today. You've had a long week, there's always tomorrow." Of course this is all bullshit because once I start, it's game on.

Half the battle is just showing up.

I have never regretted powering through a workout that I was hesitant to begin.

I'm always grateful for doing the work when I had the chance to. My reasons for wanting to skip a workout may be valid, but succumbing to comfort and status quo will only keep me exactly where I am which is just not going to work for me.

What writes our story and cultivates our warrior spirit are the *in the moment*, game time decisions that we face day to day. Some of the most successful people in the world use their work ethic in the gym as the nucleus for their life, regardless of how busy they may be.

Dewayne Johnson, a.k.a. "The Rock", is the real deal. He wakes up at 3:45am every day and does a two-hour workout before beginning work on his many projects. (Check out his Instagram if you ever need a little motivation.)

I can hear the haters now, "Well, if I had millions of dollars I would have time to train like that too." Bull shit! If that were true do you really think he would be waking up at 3:45 am to do it? No, he sticks to that routine because that's what got him to where he is today, not the other way around it.

Before The Rock grew to prominence, he was a rebellious kid, flunking out of school, and having run-ins with the law. He credits exercise and fitness as being his salvation. He was able to turn his life around by developing an intense workout regimen and work ethic.

Being motivated to outwork everyone around him provided him with the model for how to win at life. He was able to apply this work ethic to other avenues in his life, including his career. He brings the same level of discipline and intensity to acting as he does to his workouts and fitness regimens.

The same can be said for many high achieving people. **The warrior spirit lies dormant in most of us, but the few who nurture and embrace it succeed at life on all levels.**

Those who fully embrace the warrior spirit do not see exercise as something that takes time away from their life, but as something that adds value and structure from which their capacity for massive success emanates.

When you hold your time in the gym as sacred space you take control of your day. No longer are you pulled frantically in every direction, putting out life's little fires; fires that manifest themselves through people, places, and things. Instead you have staked claim on your day. From that one self-nurturing decision your level of consciousness rises and lets the world know that your time is to be respected.

Life is a mirror. The outer world that you experience is a reflection of your inner world. If you do not respect your time, nor shall anyone else. People will take from you exactly what you allow. If they know you will cancel your workout with a little pressure, then don't be surprised when something pops up every time you're about to head to the gym. What's urgent is rarely important. Save your workout karma for what's important.

You don't have to be the Rock in order to change your life with fitness. For an easy guide on what steps to take to create a fitness routine that will serve as a catalyst for your healthy style, here are three things that the fittest people in the world do.

3 Things the fittest people in the world do

1. **They view exercise as something they "get" to do rather than something they "have" to do.** Is it just coincidence that some of the most in-shape people I have ever seen just love working out? Was it the love of movement that got them there, or the results that kept them going? It is a chicken or egg question. When you adopt the mindset that movement is fun and expressing yourself physically is your equivalent to a monk meditating, then you may find yourself prioritizing the gym a little more. If you consider what the average American does after they've clocked out of work (Netflix and chill?) then it is no wonder why so many of us see the gym as a necessary evil rather than a welcomed retreat. This distinction alone is what separates the high physical achievers from the "New Year's Resolutioners" who yo-yo throughout the years, always gearing up for their next big run at a getting healthy. If you view an hour at the gym as taking away from your life, then I would challenge you to examine how much time is spent on non-nurturing behavior: binge watching TV, drinking too much alcohol, social media addiction, pointless internet surfing etc. The reality is that like begets like, and the more productive you are in one area of life, the more productive you will be in all areas. Ask yourself this: Am I where I want to be? If so, great! If

not, could your feeling of non-fulfillment be linked to inconsistency? Chances are that the two are related. So let's make a commitment that is realistic. Set goalsDo not fool yourself into thinking that you can go from 2 workouts a month to 20, but what about 8? Next month 10, then 12. You get the idea. Look for the good in exercise; inject the world with your positive energy and make friends with the gym. Any issues you might have are only as big as you make them, and sharing an experience with a room full of likeminded individuals can be powerful and transformational, especially when you find that so many others have been where you are.

2. **They plan ahead.** "An ounce of prevention is worth a pound of cure." Don't let your week just happen to you. Think about everything that might come your way. It's amazing how stress suddenly ceases to rule your life when you've anticipated a potential roadblock. For example, you know that it takes 45 minutes to commute in the evenings because of traffic. That means you must leave at 5:15 pm in order to make a 6 pm fitness class, but you're STARVING! Luckily, you spent your Sunday preparing for the week and have your favorite protein bar or trail mix in the car waiting for you so that you're fueled and ready to go. You can imagine how miserable you would be if you didn't anticipate your calorie needs and found yourself feeling fatigued. I'd bet in that moment not going to class seems like a reasonable option and is why stress the importance of preparing yourself for success. Simply bringing water and healthy snacks with you on a daily basis can mean the difference between feeling like working out, or feeling like skipping yet another one. Spend the time necessary to make yourself invincible to life's inevitable surprises and you will find yourself without a good reason to skip a workout.

3. **They keep an open mind**. It's humbling when an elite member comes to me asking for help. Often in my mind they are actually better than me at the particular movement. It's a reminder that the moment you think you got it all figured out is the moment you stop learning. The endless pursuit of knowledge if the defining factor between the great and the average. The only road to mastery is through voluntary self-effort. To be great you must drop preconceived notions about what is bad for your back, what is too much training, too little training, right supplements, wrong supplements etc. Ask, experience, and learn for yourself. Obviously I am biased toward CrossFit because, to me, it is the *most* encompassing full body training program that I've come across. However, I'll be the first to tell you that it is not the end all, be all. Even Rich Froning, 4 time CrossFit Games champion plays roller hockey and flag football on a regular basis. Don't be so stuck in your ways that you do not explore new sports or ask for assistance on movements. The best athletes in the world have coaches. Not because they can't train themselves, but because they know two heads are better than one. Simply having a discussion with someone has the power to unlock the next level of their development. Just yesterday we took the SRX staff and members rock climbing. It turned out that 3 of our coaches and one of our members were actually really good. They were able to teach the rest of us some basic techniques that showed us immediate improvement. For some members this meant skipping their regularly scheduled workout for something a little more un orthodox. However, it demonstrated to them how their CrossFit training translated directly to rock climbing and how rock climbing can help their regular fitness routine. Bottom line: take any opportunity to learn a new

skill. After you try it you will see how it applies to areas of your life you would never have considered.

Don't let a 12-Week Program Turn Into 12 Months

Peak performers have it worse in some cases because their bodies are so accommodated to hard training that in order for them to see even a 1% gain in ability requires more effort and strategy than the previous 10% in gains did.

A great example of this can be found in the workout tracking software we use at StrengthRx called Beyond the White Board (BTWB). It should be noted that I do not work for, nor do I have any interest in tis company besides being a satisfied customer.

BTWB assigns to you a fitness level which is scored from 1 to 99. Your level is assessed after a certain number of entries are made. The score is basically a ranking of where you stand compared to its very large database of users.

To put it in perspective, most people can get to a fitness level of at least 50 within 6 months of consistent training. To get from 50-60, however, takes significantly more work because now you are no longer "average" and are competing in the top 50th percentile. This trend continues all the way up to where ascending a single point from 97-98 could take an entire year of program cycling, sound nutrition, and jaw dropping discipline.

As the amount of work required increases, the people who can actually achieve it become fewer and fewer. We have athletes at the gym right now that are in the upper 90th percentile on BTWB. They are some of the most elite I have ever seen in person.

The further down the rabbit hole you go, so to speak, the realities of what it takes to achieve higher levels of fitness become more clear. At this point the need to consistently reinvent your routine, recommit to the training, and fine tune your diet become nonnegotiable.

For example, drinking 2 protein shakes a day might seem crazy to someone just starting a fitness routine until you experience your first strength plateau. Now suddenly the shaker bottle everyone is carrying around doesn't seem so foreign and the information about recovery your coach has been telling you for six months finally clicks.

At first, a beginner might feel uncomfortable in workout clothes and think anyone who grunts is a tool. They might think people only chalk their hands up before a lift for show and all supplements are snake oil.
They may have feelings towards unorthodox movements like handstands and muscle ups are just ways of showing off. However, as the beginner's curiosity peaks the judgments soon fade. It's only a matter of time before they're showing up in fresh gym gear with a shaker bottle full of protein.

To get to the next level you must accept the fact that it's going to require more from you. To write this book I had to accept the reality that another 2 hours of my already very busy day were required in order to see it through. My first reaction was the same as anyone's may have been: "I don't have the time to do this. I'm too busy". The irony of course is that here I am about to write a book on what it takes to transform one's self physically by making the time for it, yet the same voice inside my head was telling me that I was too busy!

I believe that in the current state of our evolution it is our job fight the resistance we feel whenever we think about what is required to to get from where we are to, to where we want to be; or as Steven Pressfield said so eloquently in his book, "The War of Art", "The secret real writers know that fake ones don't is that it's not the writing part that's hard, its sitting down to do it. What lies between who we are and who we're meant to be is resistant."

The warrior and the athlete live by the same motto, that the battle must be fought a new every single day. The resistance toward what must be done to transcend our current station in life is felt by anyone who's ever dared to be greater than the sum of his or her closest friends.

Whether you're an artist or an athlete it is our purpose to on earth to express our highest potential. The only thing in our way is resistance, and we must go to battle with it daily.

Once we can accept what it is going to take, resistance loses its strangle hold over our destiny. This is what Dewayne Johnson and many other high achievers realized long ago whenever they heard the voice of procrastination whisper in their ear to, "Put if off until tomorrow". The secret is to take care of today. Do your best today and let your days take care of your weeks, which take care of your months, which take care of your years.

Thinking that you will get to it in the future keeps it in the future. Speed of execution is one of the most valuable assets a person can possess. Conversely, procrastination is the killer of all potential.

Mastery vs Overload

"An individual is free only to the extent of their own self-mastery."
- Steven Pressfield

Greatness is a choice, and every day we must recommit to our vision, or fall victim to the comforts of modern life.

Perhaps on some scale this has always been the case with humans. However, to our hunter gatherer ancestors, laziness was a matter of life or death. Now, unfortunately its encouraged by the people who aim to profit from our desire for the easy road. Everywhere we go corporations are trying to convince us to let them do all of the work while we sit back and relax.

Although these modern conveniences can be incredibly useful, it's up to us to not surrender our lives over to industries that would prefer we all stay predictable little consumer cogs in their wheel of products and influence.

Watch the film "Wall E" to get a glimpse of where human evolution could lead us if we keep opting for instant gratification over process orientation.

The only road to mastery is through process. You cannot fake it or have someone else do it for you. You have to get up and decide to continue your training.

Health and fitness are learned skills that are as much of an art form as painting. The analogies are infinite because your life is your canvas.

Just as a sculptor can create a beautiful work of art out of a piece of stone, so too can you remove all the crap around the work of art that lies beneath the extra baggage you have been carrying around for years. This baggage comes in many shapes: toxic relationships, unfulfilling careers, social media addictions, negative self-talk, substance abuse, non-nourishing behavior, and so on. We remain attached to our baggage even though we know it no longer serves us, and is in fact killing us. Your baggage may seem subtle, but if allowed it will attempt to convince you of it's value while providing nothing tangible to prove it's worth.

Just as the sculptor chisels away the unnecessary stone to reveal the perfection that was always inside, so too must we drop the baggage that is covering up our masterpiece, allowing the man or woman that we know is inside to emerge.

Our chisel is our attention. What are we focusing our attention on? Focusing our attention on an area of our lives is like watering a flower in order for it to bloom. Each day we have the choice of which plants, or areas, we choose to water. If we spread our attention over too many things nothing will have enough to fully mature.

This is why we must exercise the 80/20 principle and do away with the 80% of things in our lives that cause distraction and draws our attention away from the core 20% of what really matters. Choices are abundant and if we're undisciplined we can easily find ourselves being pulled in a thousand different directions.

This is usually when people employ the "busy excuse". In other words, because they have mistaken overload for productivity, they render themselves "too busy" to take on something as vital to their life as health and fitness.

In his book, "The Entrepreneur's Blue Print", Peter Voog writes about mastery vs. overload from the business perspective. I think it applies directly to health and fitness as well.

To paraphrase, Peter says that whenever young entrepreneurs come to him and boast about how they read 52 books last year he simply asks them what is the biggest thing they learned and how have they apply it to their life? Not surprisingly, it's almost always very little. He then challenges them to read the same book 3 times, not moving from one chapter to the next until they are so familiar with the lesson that they could teach it.

That was a big eye opener for me both professionally and personally. You see, our brains are so conditioned for immediate gratification that we actually get a shot of dopamine when we complete a task. So although reading a book a week feels like you're accomplishing a lot and that shot of dopamine feels good, you're not actually making a significant change in your ability to add value to your life or anyone else's. You're overloading your brain with topics and stories across too many genres, and therefore are gaining mastery of none. Although slightly more admirable than a social media addiction, to me this falls firmly in the 80% and is another form of distraction and therefore resistance.
else

To bring this concept full circle, imagine an olympic level swimmer. How would their training routine look? Strength training? You bet. Explosivity training and Cardiovascular conditioning? A must. Not to mention lots and lots of time in the pool. These modalities are all well within the top 20% and therefore strictly regimented to continue the mastery of craft that has been honed and refined by generations practitioners.

What you won't find, however, is experimentation with crash diets, disproportional hypertrophy training for size, or any other baseless trend or method that doesn't directly serve their goal of being the best in their sport. Why should the average person care what an olympic swimmer does to stay on top? Because if we don't model our lives after those who have ascended mediocrity, become the best in their field, and tamed the inner critic, then we will continue to chase our tales; working incredibly hard and getting absolutely nowhere.

How Much Of Your Day Is Spent Entertaining Yourself?

By simply changing our entertainment to education ratio (EVE) we can begin the process of self-mastery.

We all need down time, but the day in and day out unconscious tendencies towards mindless entertainment plays directly into the hands of the media industry. Become your own gatekeeper and choose wisely what you allow to hold your attention. Don't let Hollywood, Facebook, or any other form of media rob you of your precious time, for that is a sure fire way to sabotage your potential and keep you firmly in the grip of corporate America's bottom line.

I began this chapter with a quote: "There is no other road to genius than voluntary self-effort." There it is again. To me this perfectly encapsulates the mindset of the spiritual warrior.

It's tempting for a person who spends their free time pacifying themselves on social media, television, or vacations to want to brush a lifetime of work and refinement down to a single word like "genius". This desire to label someone as "gifted" or "a natural", without giving credit to the effort that was required, is a person's way of disguising the justification of their unrealized dreams in a pseudo compliment.

This ideology implies that only a privileged few is capable of achieving such a feat, and therefore lets them off the hook. However, the warrior knows that the only difference between themselves and everyone else is that they chose to educate while the latter chose to entertain.

History is filled with people who spent a lifetime mastering their craft only to be called an "overnight success" once mainstream media saw the fruits of their labor. It has been said that people only notice 10% of every 100% change you make in your life. So don't be discouraged if few people shower you with praise and admiration for starting a health regimen. Be self-referred. Go inside and reconnect with why you are doing this whenever you feel lost or unmotivated. The warrior's life is a solitary one. Avoiding hierarchical pecking orders and opinions of others is a top priority. She must keep her ambitions close to the chest and only share her goals with fellow warriors who live by the same creed.

If revealed to the wrong person, one who is more concerned with how they are perceived than by fulfilling their own life's purpose, her efforts will surely be scoffed at, undermined and diminished by those who feel threatened by her determination. If you continue to look for outside approval, then you will continue to subject yourself to the criticism of others who seek to maintain their status. Only when you become self-referred can you become a spiritual warrior.

Every day the warrior must go to battle with entertainment's lust for their attention. It's all too easy to justify and the average person will lay out convincing arguments with facts and studies on the benefits of leisure. However, the ratio must tip in favor of education verses entertainment if one is to ever achieve mastery in their lifetime.

I don't mean to sound like a scrooge who is all work and no play. I cherish my free time. I revel in recreational activities, and I am a lover of good food and wine. I am able to enjoy the pleasures of life without regret because I know it is well deserved.

The work comes first. After a workweek of focused study, exercise, super nutrition, and process orientation, nothing in the world feels better than enjoying a great meal with a wonderful glass of wine, or two, or three. However, you rob yourself of life's pleasures if by weeks end you've missed your workouts, already drank too much, and spent all your free time binge watching television.

Going out for a night on the town then seems routine and ceases to have any luster if you've not the discipline to delay gratification. Time with friends and loved ones can become spoiled if you don't take care of your days, which take care of your weeks. Deep down you feel unworthy of yet another night out. Your entertainment to education ratio is skewed and your inner warrior lies dormant, Waiting for you to nurture it and allow it to mature. True guilt free leisure can only be had when you've done the work required to progress towards your goals.

Setting Yourself Up For Success

I get it, all of this can be overwhelming. It can be a tough reality check and unfortunately this is where most people stop. They've read the book, they conceptually understand the principals involved, and they get really inspired.

Then what? The alarm still goes off at the same time every morning and you still get home from work at the same time every night. Where do we start? Sometimes the idea of a new regimen is much easier than the implementation of it, and those old familiar routines are all too comfortable and easy to fall back on after a hard day's work.

Enter preparation. This is a nonnegotiable element to your success as an athlete, professional, and all around epic human. As mentioned earlier in "3 things the fittest people in the world do", you must plan ahead.

Take food preparation for example. Winging it is a sure way to fuck up. You'll undoubtedly find yourself starving one day and revert back to old habits. The key is to plan ahead and prepare your meals in advance. If this seems radical to you then go back and re-read the section on "The Law of Accommodation" to get a grasp on what it takes to be on top of your game.

The irony, of course, is that this only seems like more work. The reality is that structure sets us free. By preparing yourself to make easy decisions you free up your mind from frantically searching for unhealthy fast-food alternatives.

Preparation comes in many forms; you can take it as far as cooking every meal you eat per week in advance, hiring a meal service to do it for you, or simply bringing your own snacks and water with you wherever you go, so that you're not tempted to cheat. This not only saves you time, but if you stick to cooking your own food it will also save you money.

We have a saying at the gym that you get trapped in the "eating out loop". Meaning you keep forgetting to go grocery shopping and therefore keep having to eat out. You end up spending twice as much money and eating half as healthy, which brings us to our next chapter.

Chapter 3
Nutrition
The definitive guide

Since the 1980s the cost of soda has gone down nearly 20% while the cost of fresh produce has gone up more than 40%. This coincides with obesity levels perfectly.

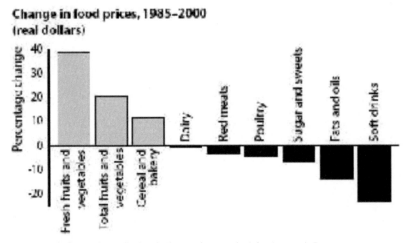

Source: USDA US Food Review, Vol. 25, Issue 3. Converted to real dollars.

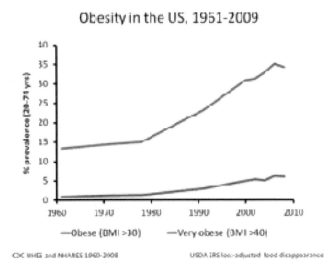

CDC NHIS and NHANES 1960–2008   USDA ERS loss-adjusted food disappearance

In his lecture, "Sugar: The Bitter Truth", pediatric endocrinologist Dr. Robert Lustig, one of the foremost childhood obesity researchers, outlines that since the adoption of the food pyramid in the 1970s nearly all the metabolic diseases that the western world suffers from have sky rocketed.

The food pyramid warned us of the dangers associated with consuming fats while toting a diet rich in whole grains and fiber as our salvation. This launched a national campaign against fat of all kinds, giving the bread industry a huge opportunity to strong arm the government into subsidizing certain crops, namely corn and soy.

You see, when we originally passed the Farm Bill back in the 1930s, tax payer subsidies were too small to influence which crops farmers grew. However, "In 1980, we introduced crop insurance subsidies of substance that began to change the ways in which farmers manage risk, and to discourage diversification," Says Vincent Smith, professor of economics at Montana State University and a visiting scholar at the American Enterprise Institute. A 2014 Washington Post article by Tamar Haspel states.

Farming is risky. These subsidies essentially made it less risky for farmers to grow grains and oil seeds as opposed to fruits and vegetables. Thus making it really cheap for consumers to buy bread and corn products, and more expensive to buy fruits and vegetables.

With all the extra bread and corn products flooding the market, advertisers had to get clever about how to keep demand high. Thankful for them the father of the modern food pyramid, Ancel Keys, graced the cover of Time magazine with his landmark study associating saturated fat with heart disease. This prompted the "low fat craze" of the 80s and 90s.

However, as Dr. Robert Lustig points out in his lectures on childhood obesity, Keys' study on countries with correlations between high fat consumption and heart disease was inconclusive, and only used the results from countries that supported his argument, disregarding the countries with high fat consumption and low levels of heart disease.

Unfortunately, it took until the early 2000s before Dr. Lustig and others would point this out. Over the three plus decades of high carbohydrate and seed oil consumption that followed, metabolic diseases reached epidemic levels.

Levels of fat in food dwindled to almost nothing. Labels advertising "Fat Free" flew off the shelves as the public was convinced the answer to their problems lied in a low fat diet. The amount of sugar in foods, usually in the form of corn syrup, sky-rocketed because the best way to make something taste good without fat is to simply add sugar.

As the consumption of fat decreased by 30% over the following 30 years, the rise of diabetes, heart disease, metabolic disease, and obesity rose nationally by more than 30%; exactly the opposite effect of what Ancel Keys' research originally predicted.

How can this be? One word: sugar. As Dr. Lustig writes on his website www.responsiblefoods.org that sugar is toxic. In a new, landmark study published in the journal "Obesity", UCSF and Touro University researchers prove conclusively that dietary fructose restriction improves metabolic syndrome.

Even today, added sugar is found in 77% of grocery store items. Adding sugar makes packaged foods shelf stable and that's good for profits, even though it's bad for you. So to get Americans hooked on "fat free", the food industry pumped us full of sugar. The World Health Organization recommends that we limit our sugar intake to only 5% of our diet; that's just 6 table spoons instead the 22 table spoons the average American consumes daily whether they know it or not.

The timing of the low fat craze, and subsequent metabolic epidemics that followed, coincided perfectly with the substation of corn and other grains by the government. Essentially making it a no-brainer for the food industry to capitalize on the public's perception of fat being dangerous, and marketing tasty fat free alternatives loaded with high fructose corn syrup.

Dietary Fat is Essential. Sugar is Not.

Don't get me wrong, we need fat in our diets. The list of health benefits is a mile long: It slows the absorption of carbohydrates in our small intestines to aid in controlling our blood sugar, produces testosterone and human growth hormone, provides us with sustained energy and acts as an antioxidant, makes our skin suppler, hair thicker and nails stronger, just to name a few.

The answer, as with most things, is to go back to basics and remember that 100 years of food manufacturing and processing doesn't nullify 10 million years of evolution.

Our hunter gatherer ancestors sure as hell ate animal fats as often as nature would allow. Now, it's true that everybody metabolizes calories differently and some people do not benefit from a "high fat diet". In order to get an accurate picture of how your body is reacting to the foods you eat; a series of blood test would need to be done. (Clinics that specialize in this can be found relatively easily.)

With that said, from my own observations, we have run several fitness challenges here at the gym where in addition to exercise the only dietary requirement is to stop eating sugar and wheat for 4-6 weeks. The results are never less than amazing. People of all ages and sizes literally transform their bodies in relatively no time at all. We had a 45-year-old woman, whose weight loss had plateaued for 10 years, drop 17 pounds in our most recent challenge. She couldn't believe her eyes when she saw the scale and that her body fat percentage had dropped 6 points.

Without specifying a low carb or calorie diet, and simply cutting out sugar, wheat, and alcohol we are seeing people achieve outstanding results time after time.

Sugar is the real threat, especially to the sedentary. Athletes handle sugar consumption a little differently, but even for the most advanced athlete it should be used as a tool for recovery. Believe it or not every form of carbohydrate you consume turns into glucose once it reaches your blood stream. Whether we are talking about table sugar, rice, or a bowl of pasta, once swallowed, your body only recognizes it as glucose.

This can be tricky if you're on a limited budget. You'll find yourself gravitating toward the middle aisles of the grocery store where the processed and packaged foods are stored. That's the system the food industry has designed. We are programmed to seek out the greatest amount of calories for the least amount money, and the food industry spares no expense to entice you with colorful packaging and claims of added vitamins.

If possible, avoid these aisles at all costs. Generally speaking, food that has a shelf life is suspect. Therefore shopping the perimeter of the grocery store ensures that the food we're buying is at least real, decomposable food.

Shopping the perimeter also means a certain amount of time will be spent cooking your own food. Aside from keeping our blood sugar down, when we cook our own food we connect with being human. Intimately working with plants and animals reminds us of the reality that industry and corporations do not feed us, nature does.

But there's no money in that, so it requires us to hack through the jungle of marketing to the truth of what we're actually eating. Even the packaging is designed to redirect our attention away from the nutritional facts and ingredients. What food companies want you to see - "made with real fruit" and "heart healthy whole grains" is alll bullshit. Like I said before, if it has a shelf life then it is suspect. We must know where the food we eat comes from and prepare it ourselves whenever possible.

Eating for Performance Vs. Weight Loss

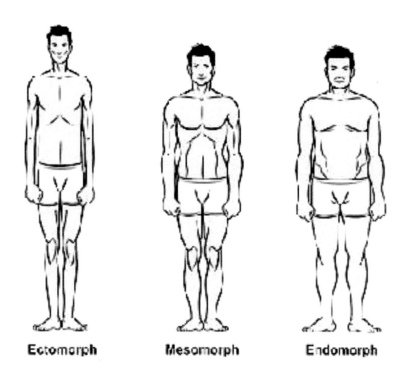

Ectomorph   Mesomorph   Endomorph

I've grown to believe that the scare of metabolic diseases, in all their many forms, has created a culture of fear towards overeating. Rightfully so in most cases. If you are indeed a sedentary person, then over consuming calories is a guaranteed path to obesity.

However, a person's "body type" should be considered when deciding on the number of calories one should consume. For example, if a person has an endomorphic body type, then he or she will most likely struggle to lose weight even with diet and exercise. Someone with an ectomorph build could most likely eat all day long, without exercising, for years and still struggle to gain weight. Mesomorphs fall in the middle of the body type spectrum, and are arguably the more universally athletic body type. How distinct these lines are is definitely up for debate. These are simply bored classifications that are in no way absolute, but do offer some insight and are worth exploring.

When you come across a clear ectomorph, you know it. The same can be said for all three types. However, there are absolutely hybrids of these body types with perhaps a dominance towards one. I would consider myself mainly ectomorph and partially mesomorph because I am 6' 4" and 200lbs. I can put on size but it is definitely a more difficult task compared to my mesomorph friends whose biceps seem to grow by just looking at a dumbbell.

On the other hand, I have it way easier than some of the pure ectomorphs I know who have been lifting weights for years and somehow, despite heavy weight training and horse like eating, never gain a single pound.

Endomorphs will most likely scoff at both of my previous examples and tell us to cry them a river, because to a pure endomorph the ratio between physical exertion to calorie consumption seems unfair; as if the exercise gods are getting a kick out of how hard people with this body type must work to see the scale move in the right direction.

Basically, it comes down to genetics. Perhaps the single most important thing to remember is that regardless of which body type you tend to resemble most, genetics do not doom nor guarantee anything. We all have the obesity gene, cancer gene, hair loss gene, muscle gene, etc.

In addition to what set of genes we inherit, our behavior throughout our lives determines which genes are inhibited and which are expressed. With sound diet and exercise, even the most extreme endomorph can become thin and the most extreme ectomorph can pack on muscle. Mesomorphs must have done something right in a previous life because as far as physical appearance goes, they got out easy, those bastards. Regardless, everyone has their own unique potential and in this chapter, we will be talking specifically about the dietary guidelines required to see that come to fruition.

Eating To Gain

Admittedly, this section comes easy to me because I fall into the category of those who need to eat for gains. I graduated high school in 2003 at 6'3" 155 pounds. Granted, high school was 13 years ago for me, but even as I enter my thirties I have managed to maintain 45 pounds of extra muscle with relatively low body fat since I initially packed on the majority of my weight at 20 years old.

I still remember the moment in 10th grade when the extent of my puniness was revealed to me in the most humiliating of ways. Like many 15 year olds, I spent my summer sleeping in, eating like total shit, and propositioning homeless men to buy my friends and I beer.

Despite my best self-destructive efforts, I made it through the summer alive and started high school thinking I was a tough guy (This probably had a lot to do with being tall). The truth of my true toughness, or lack thereof, was about to be revealed. In my hometown of Traverse City, Michigan, everyone was required to take gym class their first year of high school. This was no problem for me because I was definitely one of the strongest dudes in my class, or at least that's what my confidence of youth syndrome led me to believe.

Coach Hern's physical education class was held at 8:30am every morning. He started the year out with his own brand of fitness testing to establish a baseline for everyone. This included max attempt pushups, pull-ups, and a one mile run.

The run came first and was the beginning of a series of reality checks that I was about to experience. It took me 17 minutes to complete the mile. I was second to last only beating the chubbiest girl in class by a few seconds. My friends, who had somehow all managed to finish 10 minutes before got a good laugh out of this. "How the hell did they do that?" I wondered. Not to worry though because the pull up challenge was next. This was my chance to redeem myself and earn back my previous ranking in the pack.

There was a single file line of guys taking their turn at the pull up bar. Two spots ahead of me my friend Brandon knocked out 7. Not bad. Then Casey B., who was notoriously strong for his age, walked up to the bar. The energy in the room was palpable with everyone counting out loud as he plowed through 15 pull ups! You could tell that Coach Hern was impressed. I was up next and the excitement from Casey's feat of strength still hung in the air.

As I walked up to the pull up bar a buddy of mine in line behind me yelled out, "Let's go Schollard!" and everyone cheered. I jumped up to the bar, convinced I was about to set some kind of school record, and just hung there. My legs flailed as I ground my teeth together, but nothing happened. The room fell silent as it became clear that I couldn't do a single pull up. I was devastated. I hung there helpless for a few sad seconds until coach Hern politely asked me to step down. My friends couldn't even make eye contact with me during my walk of shame back to the locker room.

My ego had taken a huge blow, but when I reflect on my life, it's clear to me that because of that moment I became a trainer, opened a gym, wrote this book, and committed to becoming as strong as my genetics would allow. I was now a man on a mission.

Still too nervous to join gym or workout at the school, I begged my mom to buy me a weight bench. This was around the year 2000 and body building was in full force. Functional training, which I now love, just wasn't on the radar yet. At the time "fitness", especially for men, meant body building. Building muscle was a concept I didn't yet fully understand. I just knew I had to figure it out and with limited life experience, I along with most others associated getting "fit" with dieting, even though I was already a twig.

It's no surprise that I spent 2 years from the ages of 16-18 pumping iron without a single pound of muscle to show for it. I definitely got stronger but when you're 18 you don't give a shit about how much stronger your squat has gotten; you just want to look ripped. I was frustrated and wanted to quit, but a little voice in my head kept telling me to stick with it. I came across Anthony Ellis', "Gaining Mass" program which opened my eyes to the science behind size and strength. Basically, I wasn't eating enough.

I would train like an animal and eat like a bird. Something I still coach many athletes on today. Although this is a book on athletic performance, and not "how to gain 30 pounds of muscle", it is still so often the case that people spend countless hours of their life rigorously training in their respective sports and constantly fall just short of greatness only to discover that their nutrition levels are suffering, undoubtedly costing them precious training potential.

It wasn't until I was 19, 3 years into weightlifting with zero results, that I finally committed 100% to Ellis' program. For me that meant eating 4,500 calories a day in order to be anabolic (a state of muscle building). Just like that, I put on 35 pounds in 5 months.

Seemingly overnight I went from the scrawny kid in the gym to one of the big boys lifting heavy. This extra size and strength was the catalyst for all my future fitness endeavors; from competing in Muay Thai kick boxing to CrossFit competitions. I always did well because I fed my body the right amount of calories to produce the maximum strength and performance possible.

I am by no means bulging with muscle. In fact, with clothes on I look quite normal. The difference between how many calories my body is burning at rest compared to the guy next to me could easily be double simply because of my training regimen. If I were to eat like an average guy but still train like I do, I would probably still resemble that skinny 18-year-old who was working really hard and getting nowhere.

Eating to perform is not necessarily fun and definitely not easy, but anyone who takes their training seriously must commit to the proper caloric intake that will support and advance their abilities. It's about being a pro. Muhammad Ali has a great quote that sums it up perfectly. When a reporter asked him if he enjoys training hard he said, "I hate every minute of training, but I love being champion."

Pros do what it takes to get the job done. They don't shy away from eating what they must because it doesn't taste good. They see food as a tool. I'm sure even the best of the best still go out on the weekend and have a delicious meal and drinks with friends. However, day in and day out their eating is a part of their training for which they've committed to. Don't blow your chance of being great because you don't have the disciple to fuel your body.

For the average person 2,000 calories a day is plenty to be healthy and fit. However, you're not reading a book on how to be average. I want you to realize your genetic potential and capitalize on it. If you consider that our hunter gatherer ancestors not only survived but thrived in a time of feast or famine, then imagine what we can become with consistent sound nutrition and rigorous exercise. Nowadays food is hardly scarce, and if you're truly serious about becoming your personal best then you will need to consider the ramifications of eating too little.

I recommend using the popular metric of multiplying your body weight by 20 to find your ideal caloric requirements. For example, if you weigh 150 pounds then you would need to be consuming roughly 3,000 calories per day. This isn't an exact science and everybody will react differently. However, after two solid weeks of reaching your caloric quota you should be able to determine whether 20 times your weight is right for you. It might be 15 or 25 but the most importing thing is to start. Later in this chapter we will discuss the Zone diet which is what I recommend for performance athletes looking to gain size and strength.

Eating To Lose

If you lean a little more towards an endomorphic body type then the whole last section may have been a fun read, but the rules don't exactly apply the same way for you. Just as one's athletic ability may not be adequate due to their lack of muscle, it is also true that being overweight limits your athletic potential;

The ladder being a bit more obvious. However, if the goal is discovering one's unique genetic capacity then getting yourself up or down to your "fighting weight" so to speak, is the overarching objective.

Regardless if you're 20 pounds overweight or 100 pounds overweight, a sound balanced diet should be at the center of your program. In over 13 years of personal training, one of the biggest errors I see time and time again is the belief that, "This time I'm really going to do it!" to which the person proceeds to jump on a crash diet, run every day, and totally burnout within a week. Thus, convincing themselves that they tried everything and nothing seems to work. The self-fulfilling prophecy strikes again. Consistency is the secret, not just showing up to the gym and having a spotty diet. To the contrary, the diet must stay intact at all costs. Just as a skinny kid must eat 3,000 calories every day to get their weight up, a heavier person must stick to their diet every single day to get their weight down.

I hesitate to write this because it seems obvious, but here we are with all the information in the world available to us, yet higher obesity rates than ever. I've had more conversations than I can remember with clients who were doing really well for a time then all of a sudden lose track and begin gaining weight again. Only to discover that in fact they've been gradually allowing extra food in.

Snack favorites become the forbidden fruit. Despite it's consumption being strictly prohibited, the temptation to indulge mounts until reaching a critical mass. You can get away with it once or twice, but with each successive slip the inner resistance weakens until you've convinced yourself that its fine to eat them on a regular basis.

Usually ending with the person reverting to their old way of eating entirely and gaining back the weight that they had just lost. I'm not trying to sound pessimistic, but unfortunately I have witnessed this play out repeatedly and often with the same person. Only when we can be honest and open about the physiological obstacles one faces with obesity can we take steps to correct course.

Although a Paleo diet may not be for everyone, I have witnessed amazing transformations and weight loss for those who adopt it. Only a series of blood tests can determine how your body will react, or if it will benefit from this type of diet, so consult with your doctor before you start.

Here's an overview of the two main diets I recommend to my clients that, in my opinion, yield the greatest results.

ZONE/Paleo

Often I see members and clients alike showing up for their workouts with admirable consistence, yet remain physically unchanged after months and sometimes years of dedicated training. A little subtle probing almost always reviles the answer –poor diet. Not surprising really, and theoretically easy to fix. However, we are creatures of habit, and despite our best intentions we all too often resort back to default patterns.

So what do we do when given the undisputed evidence pointing to a sound diet? First, we need to get clear on which diet is going to best support our unique goals and body type (as discussed in the section above).

Next, we need to set ourselves up for success. Don't look at a new diet as a complete sea change that happens overnight. Otherwise you'll be left with a formidable void that will no doubt find you in a moment of weakness, elbow deep in a box of your favorite snack just days into your resolution.
Instead think of it as crowding out the bad with the good. For example, commit to eating a salad every day. Once that becomes the new norm try adding in a few extra glasses of water throughout your day. Once that's no longer a prob-

lem, and incorporate eggs or a protein shake for breakfast. Presto! Within a few short weeks your new diet is in full effect with no trace of that evil void.

Once you've conquered the basics of nutrition and are ready to take it to the next level, there are two diets that reign supreme in terms of efficacy and overall heath.

Number 1: The Paleo Diet

First let's talk Paleo. In a nut shell (no pun intended) it's meat, vegetables, nuts, seeds, some fruit, and no sugar. Earlier in this book we discussed our hunter gatherer ancestors at length, and the premise of this diet is based on the evidence that we did most of our evolution during the Paleolithic era.

Modeling our eating as our ancestors would have 10,000 years ago is the fast track to correcting our metabolism. In my opinion, this diet works wonders for people looking to drop weight and get healthy. The biggest reason is because there are no grains or sugar which are arguably the biggest cause of our current health epidemics.

Once you become "fat adapted", as Mark Sisson of "Mark's Daily Apple" calls it, you turn into a fat burning machine. However, I think even Mark Sisson would agree that an ultra-low carb diet isn't necessarily the best option for performance athletes. For these types of athletes, I would recommend a ZONE diet. :

Number 2: The ZONE Diet

The ZONE diet is a little trickier to navigate; it involves a calorie ratio of 40% carbs, 30% protein, 30% fat eaten in portions called "blocks". Each block consists of 9g of carbs, 7g of protein, and 3g of fat.

The number of blocks you eat depends on your size. All foods are categorized and it's up to you to pick the types of proteins, carbs, and fats you wish to eat. From there, measure them out in proper potion sizes based on the number of blocks you should be eating.

You need a healthy foundation in task management to be successful with this diet, but if you are an athlete who is exerting energy as fast as you're consuming then this diet may give you the competitive edge you need to keep performing.

The reason that I would not recommend the ZONE diet to someone not consistently training hard four or more times a week is because carbohydrates are fast energy; pure and simple. Unfortunately, our evolution hasn't caught up to modern abundance yet, and therefore our bodies are still wired for scarcity. Meaning that as a survival mechanism we store that extra unused energy (carbs) as body fat until the day comes when we need it. The reality is, that day rarely comes and the stockpile of body fat continues to build.

Personally, what works best for me is a hybrid between the two. I avoid grains, especially ones containing gluten, but because I am a coach, athlete, and inherently thin guy I maintain a moderate level of carbohydrates in my daily diet. I keep it around 150 grams a day mainly from yams, potatoes, and rice. I try to keep my protein levels north of 100g a day and eat all the nuts and vegetables I want.

If you look at ZONE and Paleo as dietary parameters, or a continuum of sorts, you can gauge which direction to lean toward based on your activity levels. For instance, if your goal is pure performance then you might want to turn your dial more towards ZONE, but if you look at exercise a bit more casually but want to stay trim, or just need to lose weight then shifting your diet towards Paleo will be your best option.

If you're like me and need to eat to perform well and recover, then you'll most likely fall somewhere in the middle.

Macro and Micro Nutrients

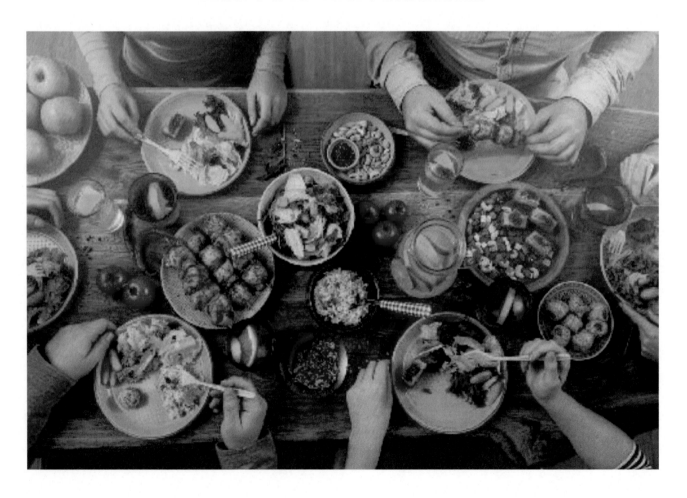

Now that we've identified which body type you are, and what your immediate aim is; for example, lose weight, build size or stay the same weight and just eat to increase performance. It's now time to gain a little more clarity on which types of macro and micro nutrients you should allow into your body.

First off, not all calories are created equal. The source of your nutrition is just as important as the consistency and amount at which they're consumed.

A macro nutrient is either a protein, fat, or carbohydrate. Proteins and carbs have 4 calories per gram while fat has 9. Micro nutrients are the vitamins and minerals found inside macro nutrient sources. For example, and egg is a macro nutrient source for fat and protein. Within fats and proteins are micro nutrients like vitamin A and E, minerals like calcium and iron, and omega-3 fatty acids.

Protein

Organic, Pastured, or Factory Farmed?

Although organic is a much better choice than conventionally farmed meats and vegetables, it's not quite the slam dunk it's been marketed to be. You would be wrong to assume products labeled "organic" are of the highest quality. It really comes down to the practices of the farm. I know this may sound like just another step you must take in the endless journey of food options, but since eating is the one thing we'll never stop doing, a little research goes a long way.

Per the USDA, organic vegetables must be grown in soil that has been free of synthetic fertilizers and pesticides for three years prior to harvest. As far as vegetables go this is about as much as we can hope for unless you want to grow your own garden, which I think is awesome if you have the time.

Meat, poultry, and eggs are a different story; this is where I'm skeptical of the "organic" labeling. There are advantages, however, especially from an animal cruelty standpoint. The USDA requires: "That animals are raised in living conditions accommodating their natural behaviors (like the ability to graze on a pasture), fed 100% organic feed, forage, and not administered antibiotics or hormones."

All great stuff as long as the farmers actually commit to these practices. From a nutritional standpoint, the argument for organic is a little less compelling.

According to a 2012 publication by Harvard's Medical School,

> "Researchers discovered very little difference in nutritional content, aside from slightly higher phosphorous levels in many organic foods. Organic produce did have the slight edge in food safety, with 30% lower pesticide residues than conventional foods. Organic chicken and pork were also about a third less likely to contain antibiotic-resistant bacteria than conventionally raised chicken and pork. However, the bacteria that causes food poisoning were equally present in both types of foods."

So, it appears that the main upsides with organic are better treatment of animals and lower levels of pesticides. This is a big plus! However, pasture raised animals, in my opinion, are the optimal choice. This is where we see the highest levels of nutrition, the least amount of animal cruelty, and the most environmentally sustainable farming practices.

You know it, I know it, and the vegan knows it. We need protein. Can we live without it? Sure, but I wouldn't recommend it. Especially to the aspiring athlete, the science is just too conclusive. Are there some vegan fitness anomalies out there? Of course, but the exceptions make the rule.

Proteins are the building block of life. Although we can find protein in other sources than meat, it almost always involves the over consumptions of carbohydrates to reach adequate levels. It's widely accepted that for your body to reach peak recovery you need to eat about one gram of protein for every pound of body weight.

In this case, and in order to expedite performance and recovery, the path of least resistance is through animal protein. Morally however, it's a different matter. I'd be lying if I said I didn't feel guilty consuming animals. I do, and it's something that I have to question myself on constantly. I love animals and nothing makes me angrier than seeing the innocent mistreated. Growing up I had pet dogs, cats, birds, a horse, guinea pigs, even pet rats at one point. So, when I devour a chicken carcass I feel the pang of guilt thinking of how that bird got to my table.

I would imagine some do not have an issue with it at all, but I've reconciled mine with a few "best practices" when consuming animals: Not all meat is the same. As discussed earlier, for me to feel comfortable consuming meat on a regular basis, the animal had to have been out in a pasture, under the sun. foraging and eating the bugs and grass that its own shit helped to fertilize for its entire life.

Not just the first 6-12 months of its life before being shipped off to the feed lot to get fattened up with grains and slaughtered. The alarms about meat being inflammatory and bad for us are nearly all from research done with factory farmed, grain-fed animals. Foreign feed from soy and corn combined with incredibly tight and unsanitary living conditions, multiply the chances of making the animal sick.

Since sick cows are bad for business, antibiotics usually come blended right in with their corn and soy feed. These factory farmed animals are without any room to roam or exercise their legs, which make them incredibly weak to the point where they often can't support their own body weight.

There is no money in scrawny livestock. To accelerate maturation, animals are pumped up with heavy doses of hormones before heading to the chopping blocks .

Organic, grass fed pastured animals, on the other hand, are at least able to spend their lives outside contributing to the ecosystem from which they feed, like all sentient beings should. Even though its time on earth will come to an end sooner than natural causes would've determined, its life will have been taken humanely and with gratitude from the people who choose this kind of farming practice over factory.

Just like with red meat, "Cage Free", "Free Range", and "Organic" Poultry can be misleading. Hear me out before you roll your eyes. According to the USDA, poultry is considered "Free Range" when the barn in which the birds live has a

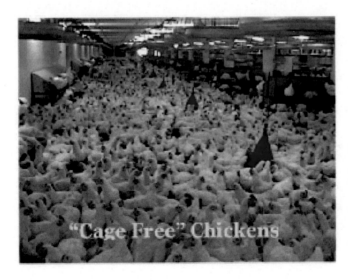
"Cage Free" Chickens

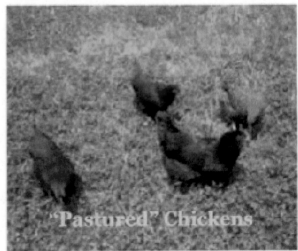
"Pastured" Chickens

single access port to the outside, no bigger than a dog door. So, even though the birds could technically go outside, the reality is that they don't. Their entire life is spent indoors with a steady supply of corn and soy feed, so why would they bother venturing out into the unknown?

By the way, if that corn and soy feed just so happens to be organic then guess what? The birds are organic.

The "Cage free" label has no regulations or standards. It simply means the hen was not raised in a battery cage, but still raised in a jam-packed unsanitary CAFO (Concentrated Animal Feeding Operation).

A study conducted by researchers in Penn State's College of Agricultural Sciences has shown that eggs produced by chickens allowed to forage in pastures are higher in some beneficial nutrients. Paul Patterson, Professor of Poultry Science writes:

> "The chicken has a short digestive tract and can rapidly assimilate dietary nutrients. Fat-soluble vitamins in the diet are readily transferred to the liver and then the egg yolk. Egg-nutrient levels are responsive to dietary change." The study also reported that "Other research has demonstrated that all the fat-soluble vitamins, including A and E, and the unsaturated fats, linoleic and linolenic acids, are egg responsive, and that hen diet has a marked influence on the egg concentration."

These benefits were not found in caged nor cage free birds. Despite it's friendly sounding label, "Cage free" does not mean cruelty-free. According to humane-societyy.org, "Both caged and cage-free hens have part of their beaks burned off, a painful mutilation." Although Cage free birds have a significantly better quality of life, due to being able to lay their eggs in a nest, run, and spread their wings, there are still more tangible benefits to eggs from "pastured" birds. For example, pasture raised birds can roam and forage outside all year- round, eating bugs, absorbing the sunlight, and re-fertilizing the earth. These conditions help the birds develop a natural robust immune system, unlike factory farmed birds that must be fed antibiotics from birth to stay healthy.

This all may sound corny and perhaps a little on the hippy side, but as with anything in life the more information we have the more likely we are to make better decisions. A fully conscious person considers where his or her food is coming from and the effects of their choice to purchase from one producer or the next. It is to avoid taking responsibility to think that the source of the meat we consume doesn't matter.

The days of offering a portion of every kill to the gods may be over for most of the world, but we can still show respect for nature by choosing to consume only the meat from animals that are healthy and unharmed.

If the moral aspect doesn't sway you, then consider something a little more objective —the treatment of livestock and the nutritional value of its meat go hand and hand. As with eggs, cows that were able to roam grassy pastures have a very different nutritional profile than factory farmed cattle.

Depending on the producer, grass-fed beef most likely contains less total fat than grain-fed beef, but a lot more Omega-3 fatty acids and CLA. Both are very beneficial to our health. Even though this way of eating is slightly more expensive, I can think of no better way of voting with your dollars than to opt for "grass fed" and "pastured" when buying protein. Change the direction of the farm industry by increasing demand for better protein. It's no longer true that, "You are what you eat." A more accurate statement would be, "You are what you eat, eats."

Dietary Fat

Animal fat such as butter, cream, lard, eggs, beef (grass fed of course) and even coconut oil are a few examples of saturated fats. You'll notice that all of these fats remain solid at room temperature. The reason for this is simple; a fat is considered "saturated" or "filled-up" when the chain of carbon atoms is fully "saturated" with a hydrogen atom, thus blocking oxidation, allowing no room for rancidity to take place, and making it "shelf stable" or "solid". That's it; not because it was created in a lab by a bunch of mad scientists plotting the end of mankind (although the demonization of it by current conventional wisdom would have you thinking otherwise).

It's actually some of the most naturally occurring stuff out there. Especially compared to some of its competition. Yes, I know what you're thinking... "What about cholesterol??"

Well, let's not forget that only about 25% of the cholesterol in your body actually comes from your diet; the remaining 75% is produced in the liver and secreted into the blood stream when necessary. Although saturated fat raises LDL ("bad cholesterol"), studies prove that it also raises HDL ("good cholesterol") too, which is essential to your cognitive and physical health.

So before you carve saturated fats out of your diet, keep in mind that according to scientist Dr. Loren Cordain, author of The Paleo Diet, over 50% of the calories consumed by our hunter-gatherer ancestors came from saturated fats found in animals. That means that for nearly a quarter of a million years of evolution we ate saturated fats.

Therefore, I find it a little absurd to suggest that suddenly the human body is incapable of metabolizing them, subsequently causing heart disease, obesity, high cholesterol, and you name it. Are we to believe that these complications have arisen, exclusively, from eating animals? No way. I mean, it couldn't possibly be from processed/bleached flour, grain, high fructose corn syrup, puffed wheat, genetically engineered crops, and hydrogenated oils, could it? C'mon, that would just seem silly, right? Those billion dollar multi-national corporations would never sell us toxic products, right? Ha.

Okay enough on that. FYI, watch the documentary "Food Inc." if you haven't already. It's a masterful depiction of the current state of our food industry.

Not all saturated fats are high in cholesterol however. Take coconut oil for example; coconut oil is a medium chain triglyceride (MCT), meaning it absorbs quickly in the body and doesn't stick to the walls of arteries like some longer chain fatty acids might do. Coconut oil is really proving itself to be a miracle food. Not only does it provide all the antioxidant health benefits of saturated fats from animals without the potential down side, but recent studies are revealing anti-cancer affects as well.

It is also being shown to regulate blood sugar by slowing the absorption of sugar in the small intestines as well as promoting a healthy digestive system. Brain health and other cognitive functions are also improved by consuming coconut oil on a regular basis. Check out these videos on ihealthtube.com for some great information on coconut oil and all its benefits.

As with almost everything, moderation seems to be the answer. We can't gorge on bacon and cheese all day just like we can't continue to follow an out dated food pyramid that has been debunked. The belief that eating fat will make you fat simply isn't true. Fat is a slow burning energy source and when consumed in moderate to high amounts, in the form of MCTs or medium chain triglycerides, can turn the body into fat burning mode, or ketosis.

Ketosis is a state that occurs as the liver's glycogen stores, depletes, and converts fats into ketone bodies. Like glucose, ketone bodies can be used for energy by nearly every cell in the body. In some cases, it can serve as an effective dieting strategy for weight loss.

Since animal proteins and fats are just about synonymous in nature, it was vital for the body to evolve with the capabilities of using two energy delivery systems —one from fat and one from the more widely known carbohydrate.

When we would make a kill and consume the meat of an animal, we were getting both proteins and fats which could sustain us without the need for carbohydrates on a regular basis. Fats absorb much more slowly than proteins and carbohydrates. This meant reliable energy production during a time when carbs were in limited supply and fats were the dominant energy source.

It's reasonable to assume that most of our hunter gather ancestors were in a year round state of ketosis. Combine that with the fact that fat has over double the caloric value of carbs and proteins, and it's no wonder why the smell of fat burning on the grill still lights up our appetite the same way it has for a million years: it means energy, satiation, and community.

Fat is essential. In fact, it's so essential that there are serious consequences if one decides to limit its consumption. The medical condition of protein poisoning is a form of malnutrition from inadequate fat intake. Although rare, I believe it highlights the importance of fat to our body. Fat primes our GI tract and gets us ready for digestion, and is crucial in maintaining a healthy digestive system.

Let's Take a Deeper Look at Cholesterol

The inputs from cholesterol, saturated, and polyunsaturated fat molecules are all required components of healthy digestion. Cholesterol, along with having its physiological importance in the maintenance of skin, production of testosterone, and other hormones; as well as bile acids is a necessary part of our organs' membranes.

In infants, the absorption of cholesterol from breast milk is vital to the development of the brain and the central nervous system. In fact, 1/5th of the mass of our brain is cholesterol, and acts as a transport molecule by passing through the blood-brain barrier to deliver nutrients.

Cholesterol is believed to block our arteries, cause atherosclerosis, stroke, and other vascular complications. In the general sense this can be true. However, there is way more to the story than the simplistic classification of "good cholesterol" (HDL) and "bad cholesterol" (LDL) which would leave one mostly thinking cholesterol is bad news all together.

Recent studies are revealing that cholesterol is found in our arteries because it acts as a patch to repair the lesions left by inflammation, usually caused by excessive glucose or trans fats in the blood stream. Once the inflammation goes away, so does the cholesterol patch. The problem is that given the realities of the standard American diet (SAD) the inflammation does not simply go away. Therefore, the cholesterol patch continues to build up, restricting arterial blood flow and potentially causing a clot, even though cholesterol was simply doing it's job.

The excess presence of glucose and trans fats in our modern fast-food, pre-packaged, frozen, and boxed meal diet has thrown our homeostasis off. In an effort to find fast answers, medicine has tagged cholesterol as the scape goat to many of our health problems. However, we can take back control of our health by understanding that arterial cholesterol is symptomatic of other inflammatory bio markers like high glucoses and trans fat consumption. Opting for high quality meats and vegetables, cutting out sugar, and staying away from junk food could be the easiest and most effective preventative measure against excess cholesterol.

However, that's not the whole story. The amount of cholesterol in our blood stream at any one time is carefully regulated by our liver. We produce around 1,000 to 1,400 milligrams of cholesterol a day, compared to the USDA recommended daily dietary intake of 300 milligrams. The amount of cholesterol the liver produces adjusts depending on the amount of cholesterol we consume. So if you eat less you produce more, and if you eat more you produce less.

In fact, only about 25% of the cholesterol we consume is absorbed by our bodies. Often people suffering from high cholesterol levels have inherited genetic problems.

HDL VS. LDL

Ever wonder what HDL (High Density Lipoproteins) and LDL (Low Density Lipoproteins) are? Believe it or not they are not actually cholesterol. They are transport molecules for cholesterol; the vehicles that move cholesterol around the body for all its roles and responsibilities.

HDL, (the one everyone loves) is recognized for transporting cholesterol back to the liver after the body is done using it for all its impressive jobs. Once it is back in the liver it is secreted as bile to aid in digestion. Although LDL is the red headed step child of the two, it has a very important job as well. Whereas the HDL brings used cholesterol back to the liver for secretion, LDL has the duty of transporting cholesterol, produced from the liver, to the tissues of the body.

Cholesterol has an extensive list of jobs and responsibilities within the body, and LDL has the thankless responsibility of getting it to all the necessary places to fulfill these duties. The old belief was that the big pillowy Low Density Lipoproteins (LDL) were the cause of arteriosclerosis and heart disease. Current research now reveals the big LDL from dietary fats has little to no effect on the disease.

In fact, it's the smaller sub particles of LDL (which are formed mainly as an effect of eating refined carbohydrates) that are causing inflammation in our arteries, leading to heart disease. This is yet another piece of evidence pointing us to the realities of poor modern nutrition, and back towards a time when eating meant an exchange of energy for calories.

Carbohydrates

After reading the previous section you might wonder why one would even need carbs? My answer is; carbohydrates are a tool that should be timed correctly and adjusted daily depending on activity levels. Carbohydrates are energy, pure and simple. Early in our evolution food was scarce. Eating carbohydrates usually meant climbing a huge tree and getting stung a few times for a honey comb, or foraging for hours to finally come across a ripe fruit.

Despite rows and rows of glistening apples, bananas and oranges in our super-markets today, the chances of actually coming across such a fruit in nature was incredibly rare. So, when that happened, our body quickly put all those glucose calories to work, giving our system a recess from creating ketone bodies.

If by some small chance our hunter-gather ancestors had a big score and ate until they're muscle and liver's energy stores (glycogen) were full, the hormone Insulin would make a tiny deposit in their fat cells with the remaining unused glucose calories. This would certainly be burned off by the next day or so. It's an awesome system of energy conservation that has gone completely out of whack from the amount of carbohydrates we're now consuming.

Tubers and root vegetables were also rare. Going through the process of making them edible often burned more calories than they contained; it was worth the effort though because of their fiber and mineral content. As omnivores, we need a plethora of food sources to keep our bodies functioning properly. Although it is possible to survive without carbohydrates, more often than not the plant from which we derive the macro nutrient "carbohydrate" from also provides the micro nutrients we rely on as well.

However, this generally pertains to living natural carbohydrate sources like vegetables and even grains, as long as they're not bleached out. In fact, as the soluble fiber we consume by eating living carbohydrates makes its way through our digestive tract it begins to ferment. This fermentation process in our gut is one of the most beneficial reasons to consume living carbs along with getting key vitamins and minerals.

The process of fermentation is one of the oldest methods of enhancing nutritional properties, preserving foods, and even creating new nutritional benefits from foods, including feeding our gut flora. Gut flora is the microbial environment living in our GI tract that accounts for about 70% of immune system. The microorganisms that reside in our gut flora outnumber the cells in our body 10-1 so it is in our best interest to keep them happy and feed them what it wants.

Bread: To Eat, or Not to Eat?

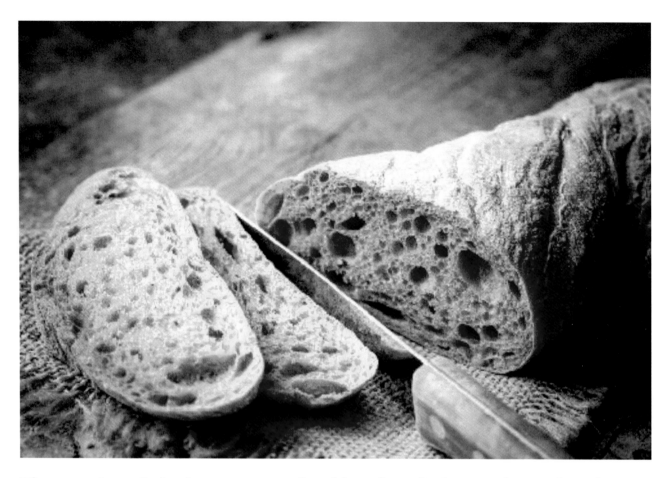

The question of whether someone should eat bread often surfaces when discussing the role of carbohydrates in our diet. Humans have been consuming bread for over 6,000 years. We've had an affinity for the stuff ever since the first person got the idea to mix ground up wheat flour with water and bake the doughy byproduct.

The smell alone instantly reminds us of home even though most of our parents probably didn't bake it. To paraphrase Michael Pollan from his book "Cooked", real estate agents often recommend baking a loaf before showing your house to fill the air with the nostalgic smell of fresh baked bread.

Unless you are fortunate enough to live near an authentic baker, chances are the bread you're eating today is a far cry from what humans were surviving, thriving and even writing poetry about up until the last century. The reason is quite simply because baking bread is hard, at least the traditional sourdough way.

It's way more of a craft than a simple process of measuring exact ingredients together in a bowl. Real bread, and the cultures that make it delicious, is a living breathing thing that needs coaxing into fruition. Because of this, baking bread at home became less and less realistic as Americans began to work more hours in a day. As with any commercialized convenience, big corporation jumped at the chance to pick up the slack and do the work for us.

This is where it all went to shit. See, plain sourdough, or any bread for that matter, only requires a few ingredients, but it's the chemistry of these ingredients that make it something to celebrate. You can't live off of flour alone, but you can live off of bread.

 In the beginning all bread was sourdough. It was made by letting unbleached flour and water collect bacteria by sitting out in a bowl under a cloth. Eventually the mixture would collect the appropriate airborne bacteria required to create the wild yeast cultures. A fermentation process would begin and the various bacteria in the culture would raise the acidity levels, creating that distinctive tangy taste in baked sourdough as well as improve its resistance to mold and staling.

True sourdough is much more nutritious than what most of us consider to be bread today. The unbleached flour and slight fermentation slows down the carbohydrate absorption rate into the blood stream, thereby giving it a lower glycemic index than the sliced loaves we're accustomed to nowadays.

This helps keep insulin levels down by not raising blood sugar levels. The problem with the Wonder Bread brands of today is the use of bleached flour, commercial single strain yeast, and added sugar for improved flavor.

Wild yeast takes time and is hard to create at mass scale. Commercial yeast on the other hand is much more predictable and can easily be replicated to produces huge quantities in a short period of time to satisfy the demands of a carb addicted culture. Unfortunately, the big corporate advertising dollars worked, and the majority of Americans now picture perfectly cut, bleach white slices in a plastic bag when they think of bread. It may satisfy our carb fix but does more harm than good by leaving us calorically rich but nutritionally poor.

My feeling is that bread, in and of itself, made the old-fashioned way with the best ingredients on earth absolutely falls into the "sensible indulgence" category. However, the commercialization of it has rendered the stuff harmful to our health and is a major reason we are experiencing metabolic epidemics in the developed world. Although we all love it, I would recommend taking a very close look at the source and the ingredients before purchasing.

In his book "Grain Brain" neurologist David Perlmutter, MD rattles our conventional beliefs about the consumption of carbohydrates in general, and grains in particular. He reveals clinical evidence linking the over consumption of grains and sugars to dementia, Attention Deficit Hyperactive Disorder (ADHD), chronic headaches, depression, and scientifically proves how our mind and body thrive from fat and cholesterol.

He argues that by simply removing grains from our diet we can undo the majority of the health problems the modern world faces. By eating a diet rich in fats and cholesterol we actually activate our "smart genes" and spur the growth of new brain cells at any age —a feat that was widely considered to be impossible for adults until the early 2000s.

This argument builds on the information outlined in the previous section about how cholesterol, or more specifically LDL, is only harmful in its sub particle forms which are developed from glucose, not cholesterol. High carbohydrate consumption undeniably raises triglyceride levels and oxidizes LDL causing inflammation, an undisputed cause for heart disease. Despite what Big Pharma has implanted into our heads, to this day there is no sound medical evidence that elevated cholesterol has any link to heart disease. Inflammation on the other hand is a huge biomarker for heart disease, and what causes inflammation? High carb diets.

What it boils down to is understanding carbohydrate's effect on the mind and body. I mentioned in the beginning of this section that carbs should be looked at as a tool. What I mean by that is if you're an athlete recovering from an intense training session then sports science points to around 30-50 grams of carbs as the optimal amount needed to replenish your glycogen levels, especially if you intend to train again that day.

For athletes, 200-300 grams of carbohydrates a day from high quality sources like quinoa, yams and sprouted rice are perfectly legit for maintaining high levels of performance. However, if you are spending the majority of your day sedentary and/or trying to lose body fat, then triple digit daily carb intake will have an extremely different effect on you than someone who is in peak physical condition.

Inflammation and high triglycerides are much more of a threat for a sedentary person because their metabolism is low and their body is in a constant state of "storage mode". High carbohydrate consumption combined with extremely low activity levels is a recipe for obesity and type II diabetes, two completely unnecessary and avoidable diseases that are the result of the over consumption of carbohydrates.

Carb Cycling

Body builders have known this trick for awhile: to stay lean yet not lose any muscle, carb cycling is the optimal solution. Science is now backing it up saying not only is it an effective way to look great, but has quantifiable health and performance benefits as well.

Carbs should be looked at as a tool to increase performance and recovery. Not the size of our mid-section. Let's clarify what I mean by that and how you can effectively harness the power of carbohydrates without accumulating any unwanted body fat.

Think of the amount of energy stored in your muscles, known as glycogen, as a bucket of water. When we train hard and exert energy the levels in the bucket drop. When we rest and consume carbohydrates the levels fill up again. So the idea of cycling your carbohydrate intake really boils down to only consuming them during periods of high exertion.

For example, today is a training day for me, so I'll eat an extra 40 grams of carbs a couple hours before my workout, and another 40 grams immediately after. This only refills my bucket so to speak, without spilling over into fat storage. If on a non-training day I roughly consume around 150 grams of carbs, on training days I will consume 200 grams, 40 before the workout and 40 after.

This works well for a few reasons:

1. It keeps my blood sugar levels low on days I'm not exercising. This in turn keeps my body fat levels low because there isn't any extra glucose floating around in my system to be stored for later.

2. It promotes higher levels of growth hormone (GH). Growth Hormone and insulin have an inverse relationship. When one is up the other is down. Insulin is released when we consume carbohydrates. So, If I keep my carb intake limited to pre and post workout, I am able to reap all the benefits that GH has to offer. The only time GH and insulin are present together is immediately following a workout when IGF-1 is released (insulin like growth factor -1). This is why consuming carbohydrates immediately after a workout is so effective for recovery. It's a perfect storm of hormones that usher glucose directly to the muscles without spilling over into body fat. *More on hormones in the next chapter.

3. It breaks my body's dependency on glucose for energy. On non-training days when carbohydrate consumption is low, my body has to mobilize fat cells to keep up with energy demands. If I satisfy those demands with a high daily dose of carbohydrates, then my body will continue to rely on that form of immediate energy, thus subjecting myself to mood swings and lethargy if I don't get my "fix". Adapting my body to work well on low carb/non training days stabilizes my energy levels and keeps all my systems running smoothly.

A 2016 study conducted by the American College of Sports Medicine titled, "Enhanced Endurance Performance by Periodization of Carbohydrate Intake: "Sleep Low" Strategy" found that athletes actually increased their performance by stopping their carbohydrate consumption after 4pm and by "sleeping low".

The study was conducted by splitting 20 athletes into two groups. Both groups ate the same amount of carbohydrates and trained using the same regimen. The only difference was that one group consumed their carbohydrates earlier in the day, while the other group consumed them evenly throughout the day.

At the end of three weeks the group that consumed all their carbs before 4pm and "slept low" saw a significant increase in maximal and sub maximal performance, with a decrease in total fat mass, but not a decrease in lean muscle mass.

To me, this study says everything I need to know about carb cycling. By going carb free for 16 hours from 4pm to 8am, it allows the body to release GH and mobilized fat storage, both of which are inhibited when blood-glucose levels are high.

Without any other dietary adjustment, simply ending carb consumption earlier in the day could have a significant impact on your health and appearance.

We Should All Be Cooking.
At Least Sometimes.

Harry Balzer, leading researcher on food and beverage trends, expert in food consulting and eating behavior, as well as vice president of the NPD group points to a steady decline in America's propensity for cooking.

The bottom line he says is, "Americans don't want to cook, the evidence is clear we want fast and easy food. Thirty years ago 70% of the population cooked their dinners. Today it's below 60%." This may not be an eye popping number at first glance, but a trend that will no doubt continue according to Balzer. He points out that Americans are still very interested in getting healthy, yet as a whole fail time and time again to achieve the desired outcome.

This stems from a lack of measurable benefits one gains by making a decision to cut out the latest single ingredient that everyone is blaming for our problems. For example, he poses the question, "What's the immediate benefit you feel when you opt for sugar free soda? Nothing. What's the first thing you experience when you cut down on sodium? Again, not much." The lack of immediate gratification keeps us from sticking it out long enough to experience any real results if there were any to be had at all.

We're quick to latch onto the latest "save all" health measure, and also quick to ditch it once we realize we feel the exact same as we did before. In other words, we continue to buy into the demonization of isolated food groups like fat, carbs, cholesterol, sodium, caffeine etc. only to discover in a generation or so that it really isn't the killer it was made out to be.

We're convinced the answer is somewhere out there when really it's been in your kitchen all along. I suppose its human nature to think that the times we happen to live in are the most knowledgeable, most evolved and most thoroughly researched. However, just as current research continues to debunk past beliefs, one can only assume that even our research will too be debunked at some point.

What has always withstood the test of time is the undisputed value in good ol' fashioned home cooking. Even if you happen to have a couple of carb heavy meals throughout the week you're still way better off than if you were consistently eating out, especially if you're the one doing the cooking. Eating out for every meal is a guaranteed way to spend twice as much money and eat half as healthy.

Let us not forget that restaurants, despite their advertising, are in business to make a profit. That usually comes at the sacrifice of high quality ingredients, for the most part. Of course there are exceptions, but for the vast majority of us the day to day restaurants we frequent are designed to get you in and out fast.

It seems crazy to me that so many people are reluctant to accept the correlation between pre-made, packaged, subsidized and refined food consumption with obesity, heart disease, diabetes, arteriosclerosis and so on. To me, this is anything but coincidence. The relationship between these diseases, the decline in cooking and the increase in fast/processed food consumption is too obvious to ignore.

I know what you're all thinking; "I don't have time to cook" right? Fair enough. I used to think that way as well, but then I got a little more specific on how much time was actually needed to cook for the week. The biggest time commitment is the prep; let's say that prep takes around 30-45 minutes for most dishes. This includes rinsing, chopping, seasoning and clean up. Once the dish is cooking, required attention needed is reduced to a couple of check-ins until it's complete.

The same can be said for "fast food" though; the time spent driving to the restaurant, waiting in line and waiting for your order to come up equal about the same time it takes to just cook your own food. Really it's a pattern one must establish, but once the routine is set it's actually a very enjoyable experience.

For most people, Sunday seems to be a great time to prepare their meals for the week. With a few simple recipes you could easily delight yourself with a stack of delicious and healthy meals in your fridge, ready to go. At my home, one of our favorite devices is the crock pot. With 10-15 minutes of chopping and seasoning you can toss a whole pastured chicken in there before noon and by the evening there's a fantastic pot of nutritious food waiting for you. Recipes abound online for delicious stews and braises. The crock pot can make enough to last for days and cleanup is a breeze. Honestly, a nice crock pot and maybe a big stir fry is enough food to feed me for the week, and all for less than the cost of one day eating out. It may seem like a lot of extra work at first, but once you've made it a routine you'll realize the health and financial benefits of cooking for yourself.

Bottom Line:

Nutrition can be a very confusing subject. Corporations make it their mission to convince us their product is harmless, but the key take away from this chapter is balance. You don't want to be the person counting your almonds at a party, but you also don't want to be the person who takes everything at face value either. When it's time to enjoy your life and indulge then go for it without regret. Then, get right back to your program and continue your practice of lifestyle design through diet and exercise.

Remember, we vote with our dollars. We choose what the suppliers put on their shelves by our purchasing. It's simply supply and demand. If more people choose grass fed, pastured and organic meats and vegetables then more farmers will opt for those practices over factory farming. The choice is ours.

Zone diet principles with paleo diet ingredients seem to be the most effective combination of caloric portions and nutritional density. If you're a hard gainer you definitely need to be less sparing on your food consumption, but you can still use this diet model to meet your goals by adjusting food intake to around twenty times your body weight in calories.

On the other hand, folks struggling with weight loss should adjust their food intake as follows:

Men should follow a primarily paleo diet with carb intake between 100-150 grams daily, with total calories between 1,800-2,500 depending on how much weight you're trying to lose.

For women, the same rules apply with the only difference being daily caloric intake between 1,500-2,000 depending on how much weight you need to lose.

For example:

If you're an athletic female who's only twenty pounds or less over weight, then a primarily lower carb focused diet around 1,800 calories a day is where I'd start you. If you're more than twenty pounds overweight with low to moderate activity levels, then a lower carb diet around 1,400 calories a day is your starting point. Adjust the calories upward for men using the same principals.

Use This Table Below To Determine Your Daily Caloric Requirements

Level one means your body fat is between 10-14% for males, and 14-18% for females. So on and so forth. Estimate your body fat level and find the corresponding calorie target. Once you determine you calorie needs, follow the sample meal plan below that supports your target.

Body weight in pounds	Body fat levels	ACTIVE MALE	ACTIVE FEMALE
	M 10-14%, F 14-18% = 1		
	M 15-20%, F 19-28% = 2		
	M 21-28%, F 29-38% = 3		
	M over 28%, F 38% = 4		
100	1	1800	1600
	2	1700	1500
	3	1600	1450
	4	1500	1375
120	1	2160	1950
	2	2050	1850
	3	1950	1750
	4	1840	1650
140	1	2500	2250
	2	2400	2150
	3	2250	2050
	4	2150	1950
160	1	2875	2600
	2	2700	2450
	3	2550	2300
	4	2450	2200
180	1	3250	2900
	2	3075	2750
	3	2900	2600
	4	2750	2450
200	1	3600	3200
	2	3400	3000

1,500 Calorie Weight Loss Diet

Meal #	Food	Serving size	Carbs (g)	Protein (g)	Fat (g)	Calories
Meal 1	Oatmeal	1/2 cup dry	31	7	3.5	190
	Eggs	4 large	0	24	20	280
Meal 2	Mixed nuts	1/4 cup	7	5	14	160
	Protein Pow-der	1 scoop (30 g)	0	25	1	100
Meal 3	Ground beef, 85/15	4 ounces	0	21	17	240
	Sweet potato	Medium	27	2	0	114
	Spring mix salad/ bal-samic	2 cups	2	2	2	34
Meal 4	Tuna	1 can	0	22	1	100
	Rice	4 ounces	40	5	1.5	180
	Avocado	Half	7	2	7	125
Meal 5	Chicken Breast	4 ounces	0	34	2	220
	Steamed Veggies	1/2 cup	11	2	0	100
Totals:			118	151	69	1,520

2,000 Calorie Weight Loss Diet

Meal #	Food	Serving size	Carbs (g)	Protein (g)	Fat (g)	Calories
Meal 1	Oatmeal	1/2 cup dry	31	7	3.5	190
	Eggs	4 large	0	24	20	280
Meal 2	Mixed nuts	1/4 cup	7	5	14	160
Meal 3	Ground beef, 85/15	6 ounces	0	31	26	360
	Sweet potato	Large	37	3	0	163

Meal #	Food	Serving size	Carbs (g)	Protein (g)	Fat (g)	Calories
	Spring mix salad/ balsamic	2 cups	2	2	2	34
Meal 4	Tuna	1 can	0	22	1	100
	Rice	4 ounces	40	5	1.5	180
	Avocado	1/2 medium	2	2	12	137
Meal 5	Chicken Breast	6 ounces	0	45	5	340
	Steamed Veggies	1/2 cup	11	2	0	100
Totals:			125	173	86	2,043

2,500 Calorie Active Diet

Meal #	Food	Serving size	Carbs (g)	Protein (g)	Fat (g)	Calories
Meal 1	Oatmeal	1/2 cup dry	31	7	3.5	190
	Eggs	4 large	0	24	20	280
	Almond Butter	1 Tbsp	3.5	3.5	8.5	95
Meal 2	Mixed nuts	1/4 cup	7	5	14	160
	Protein Powder	30g	1	27	1	122
Meal 3	Ground beef, 85/15	6 ounces	0	31	26	360
	Sweet potato	Large	37	3	0	163
	Spring mix salad/ balsamic	2 cups	2	2	2	34
Meal 4	Tuna	1 can	0	22	1	100
	Mayo or yogurt	1 Tbsp	0	0	11	100
	Rice	6 ounces	60	7	2.5	222
	Avocado	Medium	4	4	25	274

Meal #	Food	Serving size	Carbs (g)	Protein (g)	Fat (g)	Calories
Meal 5	Chicken Breast	6 ounces	0	45	5	340
	Steamed Veggies	1/2 cup	11	2	0	100
Totals:			160	182	119	2,540

3,000 Calorie Active Diet

Meal #	Food	Serving size	Carbs (g)	Protein (g)	Fat (g)	Calories
Meal 1	Oatmeal	1/2 cup dry	31	7	3.5	190
	Eggs	5 large	0	30	25	280
	Almond Butter	2 Tbsp	7	7	17	190
Meal 2	Mixed nuts	1/4 cup	7	5	14	160
	Protein Powder	30g	1	27	1	122
	Chia seeds	1 ounce	12	4	9	140
Meal 3	Ground beef, 85/15	6 ounces	0	31	26	360
	Sweet potato	2 Large	74	6	0	326
	butter	1 Tbsp	0	0	11	100
	Spring mix salad/ balsamic	2 cups	2	2	2	34
Meal 4	Tuna	1 can	0	22	1	100
	Mayo or yogurt	1 Tbsp	0	0	11	100
	Rice	6 ounces	60	7	2.5	222
	Avocado	Medium	4	4	25	274
Meal 5	Chicken Breast	6 ounces	0	45	5	340
	Steamed Veggies	1/2 cup	11	2	0	100

Meal #	Food	Serving size	Carbs (g)	Protein (g)	Fat (g)	Calories
Totals:			209	199	153	3,038

3,500 Calorie Athlete Diet

Meal #	Food	Serving size	Carbs (g)	Protein (g)	Fat (g)	Calories
Meal 1	Oatmeal	1 cup dry	62	14	7	280
	Eggs	5 large	0	30	25	280
	Almond Butter	2 Tbsp	7	7	17	190
Meal 2	Mixed nuts	1/4 cup	7	5	14	160
	Protein Powder	30g	1	27	1	122
	Chia seeds	1 ounce	12	4	9	140
Meal 3	Ground beef, 85/15	6 ounces	0	31	26	360
	Sweet potato	2 Large	74	6	0	326
	butter	1 Tbsp	0	0	11	100
	Spring mix salad/ balsamic	2 cups	2	2	2	34
Meal 4	Protein Powder	30g	1	27	1	190
	Mixed Nuts	1/4 cup	7	5	14	160
Meal 5	Tuna	1 can	0	22	1	100
	Mayo or yogurt	1 Tbsp	0	0	11	100

Meal #	Food	Serving size	Carbs (g)	Protein (g)	Fat (g)	Calories
	Rice	6 ounces	60	7	2.5	222
	Avocado	Medium	4	4	25	274
Meal 6	Chicken Breast	6 ounces	0	45	5	340
	Steamed Veggies	1 cup	22	4	0	200
Totals:			259	241	180	3,578

4,000 Calorie Mass Gain Diet

Meal #	Food	Serving size	Carbs (g)	Protein (g)	Fat (g)	Calories
Meal 1	Oatmeal	1 cup dry	62	14	7	280
	Eggs	5 large	0	30	25	280
	Almond Butter	2 Tbsp	7	7	17	190
Meal 2	Mixed nuts	1/4 cup	7	5	14	160
	Protein Powder	30g	1	27	1	122
	Chia seeds	1 ounce	12	4	9	140
Meal 3	Ground beef, 85/15	8 ounces	0	40	34	472
	Sweet potato	2 Large	74	6	0	326
	butter	1 Tbsp	0	0	11	100
	Spring mix salad/ balsamic	2 cups	2	2	2	34
	Olive Oil	2 Tbsp	0	0	28	240
Meal 4	Protein Powder	30g	1	27	1	190

Meal #	Food	Serving size	Carbs (g)	Protein (g)	Fat (g)	Calories
	Mixed Nuts	1/4 cup	7	5	14	160
Meal 5	Tuna	1 can	0	22	1	100
	Mayo or yogurt	1 Tbsp	0	0	11	100
	Rice	8 ounces	80	8	3.5	387
	Avocado	Medium	4	4	25	274
Meal 6	Chicken Breast	6 ounces	0	45	5	340
	Steamed Veggies	1 cup	22	4	0	200
Totals:			279	252	207	4,095

Chapter 4
Exercise
Skill- Power- Speed- Focus- Control

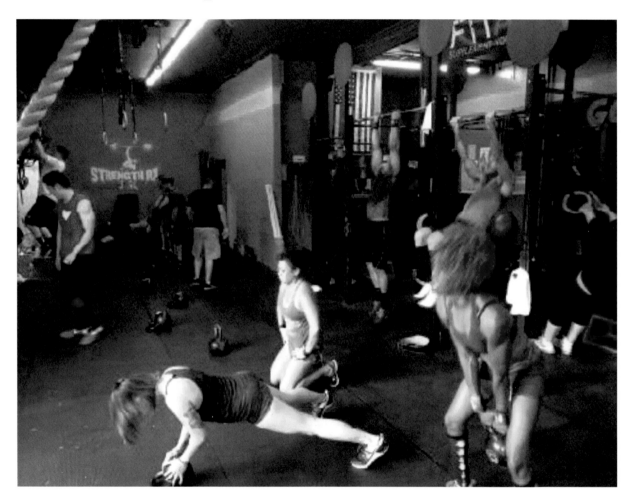

The Evolution of Exercise

Going to the gym with your friends might seem like a fairly new-age thing to do, but the ancient Greeks were actually the first to make weight training a favorite pastime. Building up the male frame in their case, was common and well regarded. Gyms were constructed everywhere for men to train in. Stone dumbbells called "halteres" were used as weights and their origin dates as far back as the first century.

The middle ages spawned a new generation of weight lifting in the form of Strong Men competitions. The methods of weightlifting were quite crude back in the day; little emphasis was placed on technique. Just a burly man with thick fatty arms and a gut would be the usual suspect in a strength challenge. These men would travel from town to town challenging the local strong men to feats of strength, much to the amusement of the townspeople. These displays of strength would include everything from lifting animals and bending metal rods, to pulling carts of stone.

In those times, the fitness scene was quite different than what we're used to today. However, there are still many types of weight lifting that have withstood the test of time. Atlas stones for example (which are incredibly heavy stone balls that people lift off the ground and place on a platform) are still widely used, and as of late, have experienced a renaissance in popularity.

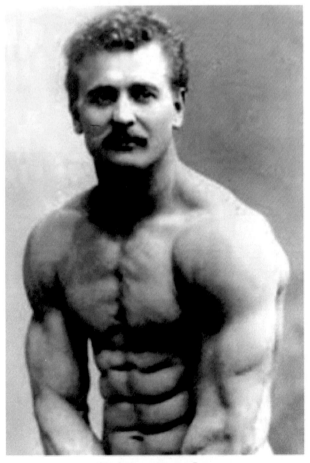

The idea of body transformation in those times grew in popularity fast as more and more people (mostly men) tested their strength abilities in ever evolving new ways. Eventually, in the 19th century, the sport of "strong men" had matured into a recognizable event that could primarily be found in circuses.

The days of bearded beasts roaming from town to town challenging the local strong men to obscure challenges

Eugene Sandow

were coming to an end as the sport refined itself. Towards the late 19th century strong men became house hold names such as Arthur Saxon aka "The Iron-Master" and Eugene Sandow, aka the Father of Bodybuilding.

This period of weight lifting represented a shift in preferences. Now it wasn't simply a matter of how much weight you could lift, it was about the human body's potential for muscular development and symmetry.

Touted as the "Strongest Man in the World", Eugene Sandow, a German man, wowed crowds with his dazzling displays of strength and muscular development. In the 1890s, he pioneered the craft of physical enhancement and symmetry through diet and weight training. He wrote many articles on the subject and created his own line of equipment that caught on like wild fire, bridging the gap between aesthetics and strength. In 1901, Sandow created the first ever bodybuilding competition and set off a craze that is still alive and well today.

Strength has been a human fascination for as far back as records go. There is even said to be a 5,000-year-old Chinese drawing depicting a soldier lifting weight as part of his training. I would imagine that the type of weight training that was going on back then in the dark dank weight rooms of the ancient world would be considered barbaric by today's standards. Then again, at the pace we're going, even the perfectly balanced barbells and polished chrome dumbbells we've grown to love over the past 100 years are being considered dangerous by newer generations gym goers who only associate working out with pulleys, cables and squeaky clean facilities.

The ever prevailing popularity of weight and cardio machines, which weigh a ton and are only intended for a single motion, dominate weight rooms. Yes, fitness is changing. Even in the heyday of Arnold Schwarzenegger's brand of bodybuilding there was still a strong sense of functional movement. In their quest for building the biggest body humanly possible, you just didn't see the stark polarization between strength training and body building as you do today.

In the 1977 documentary "Pumping Iron" which is hilarious and a must see, there are clips of Arnold training for his 7th Mr. Olympia along with fellow bodybuilder Lou Ferrigno. One clip showcases him back squatting 315 for 15 reps and in another shot he is performing a bent over row for what seems like forever with an insane amount of weight while screaming from the agony of this level of training. It was crude and far from perfect but you couldn't say the men and women of that era didn't train brutally hard with compound lifts.

In today's world of super freakishly large body builders, you'd be hard pressed to find the same level of raw functional training you did in generations passed. Instead, we humans have yet again figured out how to get the most results with the least amount of effort, and in turn the most muscle mass with the least amount of sweat. However, mass does not always equate strength. In fact, some of the strongest men and women out there look, well...pretty normal. I feel this is why many women, and some men, shy away from weight training because up until very, very recently like 2001, exercise *was* body building. The idea of lifting weights meant chest, back, arms, and maybe some legs for 20 minutes on a Saturday.

Weight training was only thought of in regards to the body part it was serving and strength in its text book definition was a byproduct of size, but rarely sought after as an end unto itself. It took a while but people eventually caught on that there was more to fitness and weight training than chest and arms. I believe CrossFit had a lot to do with this renosants in functional movements. Disciplines like Olympic weight lifting, power lifting, kettle bell training, and gymnastic were on a steady decline until Greg Glassman rocked the fitness world by introducing CrossFit: essentially combining an Olympic lift such as the clean with a basic gymnastic movement such as the ring dip. These seemingly simple movement combinations left men and women of all backgrounds on the floor, gassed, covered in sweat, sore for days, and begging for more.

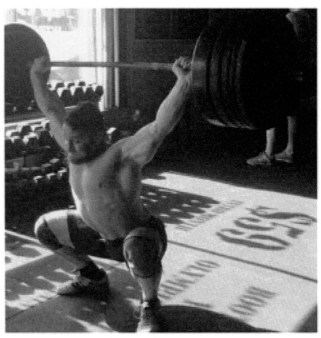

Brandon Sundwall - 255 lb. snatch

The inception of CrossFit immediately created two very different schools of thought about human movement and its applicable enhancements. At first everyone thought CrossFit was a fad, myself included. Body building forums scoffed at the cultish craze this new phenomenon was generating, and immediately wrote it off as bullshit and a great way to get hurt, but little else. However, slowly but surely the brand caught on and countered the accusations of it being dangerous by pointing out the disproportionate training regimen of the common bodybuilder.

CrossFitters redefined fitness as, "Increased work capacity across broad time and modal domains." instead of some biological Darwinian definition you'd find in the dictionary. They praised performance and using your body dynamically in pursuit of athleticism, not the engineering of sheer size for the sake of size, and mass through supplementation and training volume.

CrossFit was the first to successfully answer the call for an alternative culture to conventional weight training that was appealing to a broad audience. For the first time, in arguably thousands of years, there was a main-stream paradigm shift in the way we looked at weight training and how we spend our time in the gym.

Bodybuilding vs. CrossFit

As the flurry of articles, studies, and debates around the long term and short term effectiveness of these differing philosophies grew over the past decade, it eventually came to a head. As of this writing in 2017 it's safe to say there is a thimble full of amiability between the two warring tribes.

To the outsider this may have seemed inevitable, but to those on the inside it can still be a very touchy subject. Unless you are a professional in either sport, there is little doubt of the collision course bodybuilding and CrossFit are on. Hybrid gyms are popping up left and right with a room for legit CrossFit classes as well as space designated for conventional body building.

Personal trainers are taking their clients through a very CrossFit-like warmup, WOD (Workout of the Day), and then finishing them off with cable flies and bicep curls. Even 5 years ago you would have at least been heckled for tainting the two together.

If you ask me, this is a good thing. Although I feel CrossFit is a healthier practice for the average person in need of general physical preparedness (GPP), it won't necessarily pack on the muscle that a huge number of people still want so badly.

Don't get me wrong here, body building isn't a bad thing. In fact, to watch yourself "bulk up" and then "lean out" is pretty awesome. When taken seriously, the level of nutritional, supplemental discipline, and physiology know-how is unrivaled. Every serious body builder I've spoken with is like a freaking chemist when it comes to their body's chemistry. Cross Fitters seem to take a much more laid back approach to nutrition, but I sense a change in tides coming with that as well. The sheer interest in supplements from my members at Strength-Rx and new companies manufacturing the stuff validates my suspicion of the merging between the two.

Before CrossFit became a legitimate sport with potentially millions of dollars on the line, the go to dietary advice from most coaches was to, "Just at paleo." (Which I would still recommend to most people simply looking to tone up and be healthy.)

However, now that the pool of athletes has grown astronomically over the past decade, the refinement of its practices are evolving. In a lot of ways CrossFit athletes and their nutrition, supplementation, and training cycles are increasingly resembling that of body builders. For example, nowadays it's not uncommon to find creatine, BCAAs, and pre and post workout supplements in the Cross Fitters gym bag along with weight belts, wrist wraps and a picture of Arnold (kidding),

all of which were scoffed at not long ago. However, the raw performance increases of CrossFit athletes over the past few years are undeniable. The bottom line is that if you're competitive you're going to be at a severe disadvantage going all natural with just food as your fuel source. Apart from whey protein powder, I'm not advocating for or against over the counter supplements. It's a personal choice depending your goals. What I will say is that if you don't need additional supplements, you're probably better off in the long run without. On the other hand, if you really want to see what your body is capable of and are competitive then sure, I'd consider it. Ask your doctor and keep it legal of course.

Although I fall more into the CrossFit camp, I can see how on some level Cross-Fitters are becoming the very thing they once fought against (i.e. over training, over-specialization, and routine) Which is good, because there's no doubt that the collective awareness around proportional training and functional movement has been elevated since CrossFit hit the scene. Conversely, the periodization, supplementation, and nutritional awareness the body building camp perfected will no doubt raise the level of the common CrossFit athlete.

Even researching topics to write opposing articles about one or the other has made us all better in some sense. Where there was once a lot of uncertainty around movements such as the squat and deadlift, there are now thousands of blogs and videos from olympic level coaches online for us to devour. The resurgence of functional exercise has pooled the world's best minds and made available a wealth of knowledge once reserved for academics and professionals. Because of this, there is simply no excuse for bad trainers and coaches. Everything one needs to know about movement and exercise science is an internet search away.

Power lifting and olympic lifting have also had their critiques of CrossFit. What they consider to be pointless sub maximal contractions is kind of the point of CrossFit wods. What they can't argue with, however, is the surge in popularity these two fading giants have enjoyed since CrossFit helped repopularize their sports by incorporating powerlifting and Olympic lifting movements in their programming.

In my 5 years of owning and operating a gym that offers CrossFit as one of our main programs, I estimate that we have introduced olympic and power lifting to around 3 thousand people who had never touched a barbell, let along performed a snatch.

These people are now buying special olympic lifting shoes, watching videos online from oly coaches and in some cases even making a point to drive long distances to specific oly gyms to get some finer tuning outside of a class environment. So from my perspective, it has been a huge boom for all the related branches of weight lifting, whether they care to admit it or not.

The blending of power lifting, olympic lifting, gymnastics, body building and metabolic or athletic conditioning into one neatly packed training regimen is analogous to MMA (mixed martial arts).

This style of fighting is so dominant because you must be able to throw a punch or a kick and know how to handle yourself when the fight goes to the ground. Only those with a killer stand up and ground game are most feared. In this world, mastery of only one style is a recipe for a knock out or submission.

For the average person proficiency in any martial art puts you way ahead of the pack, but for the highly competitive world of MMA you must know it all.

Of course, there will always be purest who swear only Jiu Jitsu or Muay Thai is all you need, but the data simply doesn't back that up. Fighters with a well-rounded stand up and ground game do better.

Different exercise modalities share a lot in common with this. For example, what good are you if you can bench press a truck but struggle to run a quarter mile? Conversely, what good are you if you can run a marathon but are unable to do a single push up? As with martial arts, it's the blending of all disciplines that yields the most well rounded athletes.

On the other hand, I do believe that exercise is goal specific, and if snatching 300 pounds is your goal then bless your heart and have at it. However, for the majority of people I speak to on a daily basis, it's a combination of strength, aesthetics, health and athleticism that they are after. Therefore, the performance code as I see it is the hybridization and inclusion of all sound movement practices arranged in a way to best support your specific goals.

The Body's Energy Systems

System	Rate of ATP Production	Capacity of ATP	Fueled by
Phosphagen/ATP CP	Very High	Very Low	Creatine and stored ATP
Glycolytic	Moderate to High	Low	Blood sugar and stored glycogen
Aerobic/oxidative	Low to moderate	Very high	Blood sugar, stored glycogen, body fat and oxygen.

Have you ever wondered where your energy comes from? Or better yet, what exactly fuels your body during exercise? The answer in short is ATP, or adenosine triphosphate. ATP is the energy currency of your body. Whether you're pumping iron, circuit training or running long distances, all physical exertion requires the presence and reproduction of ATP.

The catch is, at any one point the body has very little available. So the development of strength and conditioning requires training the three main energy systems that create ATP. Each modality of training falls into one of these three.

1. Strength training

2. Interval training

3. Endurance Training

It is during the breakdown of ATP that energy is produced. Since we store very little ATP we must constantly resynthesizes it in order to continue our activity.

1. Phosphagen or ATP/CP:

Have you ever raced a friend to the end of the block where both of you took off in an all-out sprint that lasted about 10 seconds? If you're like me then you still probably find yourself doing this on occasion. It also just so happens to be a classic example of how we produce split second energy for short explosive periods of movements.

Since there's really no time for the body to recruit stored sugars, known as glycogen, to power us through this sprint, by the time our body got around to channeling oxygen for energy the sprint would already be over. So, to give the body some immediate explosive energy on hand, we keep a very limited amount of ATP readily available in our muscles just in case life demands 10-15 seconds of all out intensity of some kind.

The down side is that after 30 seconds the high-energy triphosphate (ATP) is completely depleted and converted to the lower energies, diphosphate (ADT) and monophosphate (AMP). In this pathway of 10-20 seconds worth of energy the process of replenishing ATP takes time (around 3 minutes give or take), and since it is oxygen independent (anaerobic), it does not require the use of carbohydrates or fats.

ATP solely resynthesizes in this pathway by available Creatine Phosphate (CP) present in the muscle tissue. The CP molecule converts the diphosphate back into the high energy triphosphate. After a couple of minutes you're ready to go again. This is why supplementing with creatine is such an effective way to increase muscular size and strength. An abundance of creatine in the muscle tissue increases the amount of ATP, which then increases the muscle's force production as well as prolongs the amount of time the muscle can last under maximum tension. Thus resulting in bigger, stronger muscles.

This is the dominate energy system of sprinters, olympic and powerlifters, strength athletes and anyone subjecting themselves to all out maximal efforts that are unsustainable for longer than 30 seconds. If you have ever been doing a heavy set of bench press and your muscles completely gave out around rep 5 only to find yourself able to do another set a few minutes later then you have put the ATP/CP system to use.

For sub maximal exertion lasting longer than 30 seconds we switch to...

2. The Glycolysis System:

This is the ATP pathway of boxers, basketball players, soccer players and CrossFitters for example. When you need, all-out effort lasting 30 seconds to two minutes this is the system that creates the energy for it.

During glycolysis, carbohydrate, in the form of glucose in our blood, or glycogen in our muscle, is broken down into pyruvate which are then converted by the body into ATP in a 2/1 ratio (1 glucose molecule produces 2 ATP molecules). Since this is still an "oxygen independent" system it is highly dependent on glycogen levels and/or blood glucose, which is why after a brutal circuit training or CrossFit class you're starving. Your body is trying to replenish your depleted glycogen stores.

After two minutes of all out efforts like punching a heavy bag, jump squats, or burpees, acidosis and the buildup of metabolites cause the muscle to lose its contractile ability because oxygen cannot be delivered fast enough. Usually at this point you stop as your heart rate spikes and you begin breathing rapidly as your body works to replenish APT. The good news is that ATP resynthesizes quickly in this system, and in a relatively short period of time you're ready to go again.

However, for more endurance based exercise lasting anywhere from 3 minutes and onward we recruit ATP from the...

3. Aerobic or Oxidative System:

Oxygen is the master of this domain. The aerobic, or oxidative pathway, is the most evolved and most complex of the three ATP systems. As endurance predators, human beings are no strangers to traveling long distances for food or shelter.

Any low to moderately intense activity lasting more than a couple of hours utilizes the oxidative system for ATP production. Since ATP production is dependent mainly on oxygen and not simply stored ATP, CP or glycogen, it takes much longer to fully activate than the other two pathways; once activated it produces huge amounts of ATP that can sustain energy production for hours. Think marathon runners.

This system produces 36 molecules of ATP for every molecule of glucose broken down. That's 18 times more ATP than from glycolysis. However, in order to sustain this ATP production, heart rate levels must stay below 75% of your max (220 minus your age = Max heart rate). Anything above that and you will burn through your ATP molecules faster than the oxidative system can replenish them.

The Law of Accommodation

If you haven't heard of this, you're not alone. This law states that a decrease in performance will occur if the external load does not change. Meaning, if you're brand new to exercise and you start running 2 miles every day you will likely enjoy great results for the first couple months.

This is because the physical exertion is massively higher than what your body has been used to. However, month three, four and so on will likely result in a plateau; as your body grows accustomed to the routine it will begin to undo the positive affects you enjoyed.

This happens simply because your body has acclimated or "accommodated" so well that it becomes your new normal. At this point further adaptation is no longer necessary. You see this happen when the scope of training narrows to the point where every training session is nearly identical to the one before. Whether done by fear or lack of imagination, this holds true for fitness novices and top athletes alike only varying by degree. In other words, we all have the tendency to slip into the mundane. Keeping it fresh should always be a top priority.

Variation vs. Progressive Overload

I love strength training. There you have it. Few things are more enjoyable to me then some good ol' weight lifting with a buddy. While fun and arguably important, this type of weight training can quickly turn into a leisure activity if not regulated by some kind of program.

We all know the person who reportedly spends two hours a day at the gym yet their belly seems to be growing along with their chest and arms. This usually occurs when the scope of movement reduces to bench press, rows and leg press, with some biceps and triceps thrown in there for men. The female equivalent would be something like 30 minutes on the elliptical or treadmill followed by some light dumbbell squats and presses.

A perfect recipe to stay exactly where you are. The problem, which we've already discussed is due to the law of accommodation. In the male/female cases just mentioned, their bodies have adapted to the level of training they're currently subjecting themselves to and therefore have no reason to waste precious energy adapting any further.

I would imagine in the beginning of their routines they both experienced a glimmer of hope and saw modest results. [This positive feedback seared a permanent impression in their brains that confirmed they made the right choice and set them on a track that has varied only slightly for however long they've been at it.] I've seen this scenario play out thousands of times. The problem is that as their bodies became better and better at what they were doing, the results they once boasted over faded away and left them with little more than a gym appointment.

According to the law of accommodation this can eventually have negative ramifications and leave the body less capable to respond athletically to any new outside stimulus. In other words, although the five sets of bench press and 20-minute jog provided them with immediate results in the first couple of months, after a couple years that workout can, and will impair their ability to learn and perform other movements.

We see this at the gym constantly. Usually men are the knuckle heads that come to us after years of over working their chest while their legs wither away. In these cases, we spend extra time with them mobilizing their shoulders and activating their hip muscles to get them to a place where we feel comfortable enough to have them enter our program.

We find the same shoulder/hip dysfunction with people who sit at a desk with a rounded back and forward shoulders as well. There are multiple ways to get to the same place, but the best plan is to avoid it all together.

Greg Glassman, the founder of CrossFit describes the ideal approach as "constantly varied, functional movement excited at high intensity."

Pretty right on if you ask me, especially for the people simply seeking general physical preparedness.

Exercising in a completely random way each time you work out is lightyears ahead of doing the same routine week after week. However, this isn't necessarily the end all be all. Even a routine with "constantly varied" movements has its drawbacks.

Variation can come in many forms including, amount of weight lifted, amount of time spent working out, speed of execution, amount of time between breaks, length of breaks, amount of reps and sets and of course the type of movements practiced.

Behind consistency and intensity, variation is definitely the third most important factor for getting results. However, within all the positive attributes variation offers, it can be taken too far, specifically, in regards to strength and skill training. A period of progressive overload is necessary when you're working toward a goal. Although it may seem monotonous at times to follow a program, sticking to one is essential for maximizing the likelihood of reaching a desired outcome or goal. When you begin to view strength and conditioning as a skill that needs to be practiced, you become a little more patient with the regimen.

Varying the routine can make people get a little off track. While it's true that variation is an effective way to avoid plateauing, varied doesn't mean random.

Though variation helps keep you engaged, which is definitely beneficial to the trainee, repetition is what makes you a pro. Hitting the same thing repeatedly for a period of time is necessary in order to gain mastery. The issue with completely randomized training is that the lack of a proper plan leaves the person without measurable progress.

In a "random" approach, any single workout can be great and leave you feeling sore, but if you're not working towards anything then you're likely to make more subjective decisions on your training load, depending on how you feel that day, verses what your program calls for.

Contrast that by progressively overloading the body by adding 3-5% more weight each session for 3 weeks with the same movements and rep scheme. This allows you to monitor your progress and keeps your feelings out of the decision. Based on the information you gather from your performance each workout you can then tweak caloric intake and cardio levels to help you reach your strength goals. In other words, variation should be scheduled and planned within a strength and conditioning program.

For example, if after week 3 you're not seeing any strength increases it may be wise to add a couple hundred more calories a day to your diet. Conversely, if the training program was completely randomized then you wouldn't have the data to tell if you were making the desired gains, which will most likely leave you under or over training.

More isn't always better. You could train your legs 5 times a week by preforming every squat, deadlift and lunge variation that exists and still not achieve the best results with this scatter gun approach. Without an objective standard it would be impossible to gauge where the point of diminishing returns is. Instead, I would recommend you first determine what your strength and conditioning goals are, then write out a 12-week program that progresses you towards those goals.

Within this program there is scheduled variation, weekly target numbers and rest days.

A complete 12 week strength and conditioning program is available at www.p-codenation.com

"Pure" Strength Training

Proper strength proportions are the catalyst from which the rest of your program stems from. Strength is steady and can only be achieved through consistency and patience. Once achieved, strength levels maintain their capacity for up to 10 days without training, before diminishing. Whereas conditioning levels drop within 72 hours of not training, strength training reduces your risk of injury, increases your bone density and expands your tissue's capacity.

Basically, functional strength training prepares you for life. Whether you're picking up a bottle of shampoo, a child, or a 300-pound barbell, it's still a deadlift and should be treated as such. I've seen more injuries happen to people outside of a workout. When a person is training they are focused on the lift and their form, but as soon as they've dropped the barbell or dumbbell their movement patterns fly out of the window when casually leaning over to take a drink from the fountain or bending over to tie a shoe. These simple, every day movements become risky.

Just as meditation serves as a mental and spiritual practice that develops stillness, better decision making and awareness, our hour in the gym should serve as the physical practice for our life.

You wouldn't see a monk spend an hour meditating and then scream, "Fuck you ass hole!" when someone cut him off in traffic. Yet it's common to see someone finish a deadlift workout with absolute perfect form then completely hunch their back and buckle their knees picking up their gym bag on the way out.

By taking what we learn from squatting, deadlifting, snatches etc. and applying it to the basic movement patterns of everyday life, we complete the circle of our training and put it into practice. What may seem like completely unrelated movements, in fact, only vary by degree. When you consistently train your body, and strengthen the major muscle groups of the hips and shoulders through focused compound lifts, you solidify your brains recruitment order of these muscles and reduce your chance of injury.

Strength training is a skill set that demands 100% of your attention if it is to be done correctly. As with most things, anyone can achieve 80% of their strength potential relatively easily, but to reach the last 20% takes practice. For example, to do a squat at 90% you must simultaneously ignore the hardwired alarm signals your brain sends to inform you that you are reaching critical mass, remember to keep your knees pushed to the outside of your feet, squeeze your abs as hard as possible, and avoid letting your head snap back as your body desperately searches for ways to disperse tension.

"Pure" strength training is 5 reps or under. If you're just going for size and not necessarily concerned with true strength training, then high reps and random training may work for you, as long as you're eating enough. However, that is not the focus of this book. This book is intended to make you a better, smarter and more efficient athlete, whether you play a sport or just enjoy training like you do.

When only training 5 reps and under for strength, an increase in the size of your muscles will occur, but only to a degree as your body acclimates to the new stimulus. Although a slower process, one can still put on size but it's your strength to weight ratios that will increase indefinitely given the proper programming. The reason lies in the actual make up the muscle tissue. Strength athletes tend to build muscle tissue through a process called myofibril hypertrophy, while body builders training in the 8-15 rep range tend to build muscle by a process called sarcoplasmic hypertrophy.

The difference between myofibril and sarcoplasmic hypertrophy is the way in which the tissue grows in response to training and diet. Myofibril hypertrophy happens by lifting heavier weight which correlates to a comparable increase in strength; the tissue grows by eating a relatively low carb/high protein diet. Because you're not simply injecting your muscles with hundreds of grams of carbs on a daily basis this process may take a little longer. Layer by layer your body is building dense, sustainable, and best of all, strong muscle tissue; this happens by increasing the actual number of actin and myosin contractile proteins. This type of muscle is more stable and will stick around for a long time even if training stops.

Sarcoplasmic hypertrophy on the other hand is a little easier to achieve because you are lifting in the 8-12 rep range and using up energy storage in the muscle called glycogen (see energy system #2 in earlier in the chapter). Continued depletion of glycogen levels triggers the body to increase the size of the muscles storage capacity, thereby increasing the size of the muscle. Because the reps are generally high, this type of muscle tissue is believed to not have the same strength to weight correlations of myofibril muscle tissue, and will likely atrophy as soon as high carb intake and high rep training stops.

Compound Lifts vs. Isolation Lifts

Muscular development is not exclusively achieved through machines and isolated movements. Heavy compound lifts deliver muscular strength and size with sustainable results that prep your mind and body to handle whatever life may throw at you.

Depending on your unique genetic composition, the amount of size you'll put on while performing purely 5 and under strength training will vary greatly. Heavy compound lifts such as the deadlift, squat, bench press, row, weighted pull-up and overhead press are the hallmarks of strength athletes, but for those seeking more size, a good blend of compound and isolated lifts will help boost hypertrophy.

A compound lift essentially means you are using more than one joint to complete the movement. For example, when you squat you are using your hip and knee joints to lower yourself down and stand back up. The use of multiple joints means greater overall muscular recruitment as well as higher levels of concentration.

When a lift requires multiple joints, your core must work much harder to maintain midline stabilization as you pull or push the weight through range of motion. In any lift, sharp attention must be paid to all the systems of the body. However, compound lifts have the added benefit of teaching us special awareness because they simulate natural movement patterns that force our central nervous system to engage; this then elicits our hormones which facilitate the process of building muscle and burning body fat.

In other words, the sum is greater than its parts. An isolated knee extension combined with an isolated hip extension doesn't match the benefits of a squat, and certainly doesn't teach anyone how to move correctly.

Compound lifts prepare us for the movement patterns we encounter throughout our day and translate directly to athletic application. Isolation exercises, on the other hand, train specific muscles rather than movements, and tend to over develop those muscles for pure aesthetic purposes. This runs the risk of leaving us partially dysfunctional and diminishes our athletic capabilities if not regulated.

Modern body building mainly incorporates the use of isolation exercises to achieve a desired size and shape. Although some bodybuilders may look like gods and goddesses, their bodies are often more show than go. Don't get me wrong here, I like knocking out a few sets of curls as much as the next guy, but only after I have finished the day's work of compound lifts. In fact, the people I know with the best arms never do specific arm workouts like curls or scull crushers;

they have developed their arms through compound lifts like weighted dips and chin ups. Of course, some have genetics that allow for such bicep and tricep development without specifically focusing on these areas. The same approach definitely won't hold up for everyone, including myself, but there is a lesson to be learned here: Train your body holistically with compound primary lifts and If you feel like your secondary muscles need some extra attention then incorporate isolated movements like curls, pushdowns, flies etc.

When you consider natural movement patterns and primary versus secondary muscle groups, you see an inverse relationship between what looks good and what actually serves a purpose. Deadlifts, for example, work the largest primary muscle group called our "posterior chain", which basically includes all the muscles on the back side of our bodies. Performing this exercise on a regular basis may not get you the arms and abs we all fantasize about, but it will set you up for solid and sustainable athletic development by strengthening your hips and back proportionately.

It takes discipline for the beginner to refrain from chasing the carrot and jumping into only training the glam group -- chest and arms. Patience, and most importantly, consistency will get you to the same destination in due time, with the main difference being that you won't just look strong, you'll be strong.

This type of strength based training, called functional hypertrophy, is the increased ability to create force because of greater mass, as opposed to just general hypertrophy which also results in greater mass but without the added benefit of correlating force production.

Machines vs Free Weights

Exercise machines are built with the "average" person in mind. Although they offer some interesting options for movement diversity they tend to have a one-size fits all approach. If used exclusively it's my opinion that they will stunt your development as an athlete.

A "one size fits all" approach will never deliver maximum results. You will never know your true strength levels because the blocks of weight you stick a pin into do not accurately reflect that of its free weight counterpart. To me, there's just something artificial about exercise machines.

I recently mentioned to a friend of mine how one day I would love to have a squat rack in my house. His reply was, "That would take up so much space. Why don't you just put a boflex in a room or something?" I would imagine the feeling I have towards putting a boflex in my house is much like what a drummer feels when a friend suggests they play on a drum machine instead of a full kit. Yeah, its compact and arguably better than nothing, but the reason few true drummers choose this over a real studio drum kit can be summed up on a bumper sticker: "Drum machines have no soul." Neither do exercise machines in my opinion, but since it's not as catchy I'll stick with the drum kit analogy.

The beauty of free weights is the fact that you, the athlete must wield them into place and then perform the necessary action. There's something raw and primal about this. Stepping into a cold steel squat rack and mounting the barbell atop your shoulders elicits a fight or flight instinct that exercise machines, with their padded seats and safely handles, simply fail to deliver.

An April 2014 study conducted by the <u>Journal of Strength and Conditioning Research</u> tested this theory by taking ten healthy men with experience in weight training and put them through a free weight and a machine workout to see which elicited a greater hormonal response.

For the machine workout they chose the leg press and had each male perform 6 sets of 10 reps at 80% of their one rep max. A few days later they had the same group of men perform 6 sets of 10 reps at 80% of their one rep max, with full depth barbell back squats (a tough workout mind you). During the time of both workouts the researchers placed a catheter on the participants' arms to sample hormonal levels in the blood.

The results: 25% more testosterone was present when performing squats over leg press, not surprising to anyone who's ever put themselves through a squat workout like this. More surprising was the increase in growth hormone, which was up to 200% on average during the squat workout over the leg press. When checked 30 minutes after each workout, the men still had 100% more growth hormone after squats then they did after the leg press workout.

These are remarkable findings that prove the power and efficiency of free weight compound lifts. This doesn't necessarily mean the leg press is bad, but since most of us only have a 60-minute window, 3-5 times per week to train, effectiveness is of the utmost importance.

As creatures of comfort it is in our nature to search out the path of least resistance. However, when physical prowess is our objective comfort will only make cowards of us. In the world of exercise and fitness we need to get our feathers ruffled from time to time. The body is an amazingly perceptive machine. Though it may seem inconsequential, the safety locks, padded grips and smooth gliding pulleys utilized by exercise machines put the mind at ease and the body in a state of comfort and control. This comfort and control translates to an inhibited hormonal response. As this study proves, maximum physical adaptation comes to those willing to abandon the comforts of exercise machines and step into a squat rack, prepared for an un-pleasurable experience.

Establishing a baseline with 1RMs

Another key component to training with free weights over machines is a clear, objective strength level one can establish. For example, depending on the manufacturers a 100-pound seated cable row can vary wildly from machine to machine, but a 100-pound dumbbell will always be the exact same load no matter who makes it.

Because of this you can test your true strength levels and create a dynamic, progressive program based on those results. The reason behind this is a simple lesson in sports science. We discussed in a previous section the difference between type 1, type IIB and type IIA muscle fibers. We now know that type IIB are our "fast twitch" or explosive fibers. These guys don't just activate for any-thing; that's what the type I and IIAs are for. Type IIB fibers stay dormant until the work load becomes so great that they have to activate. This usually happens around 80% of one's ability to generate maximum force, and since these are the fibers every strength/speed athlete wants more of, weight training in the 80-95% range is a must.

You can see now why testing your one rep max a few times a year in all key lifts is so important. Just winging it on your workouts will likely have you either un-der or over estimating your actual strength levels, keeping the weight either too light for significant strength gains, or by increasing the chance of injury by go-ing too heavy for the required number of reps.

In general, training above the 80% range brings you to failure by rep 5. This is why true strength training is 5 and under. Anything over that is considered bodybuilding by many. Although mass can be a powerful tool, too much will in-terfere with your athletic endeavors.

One rep max or 1RM testing in all key lifts such as the back squat, front squat, deadlift, bench press and overhead press is a catalyst for your programming. In my experience the best strength training is done by creating set and rep ranges based off of your 1RM. For example, 5 sets of 5 reps at 75-80% of your 1RM, 8 sets of 3 reps at 80-85% of your 1RM and 10 sets of 2 at 80-90% of your 1RM are common training volumes at our gym and all challenge the APT/CP path-way in different ways in order to deliver the maximum gains in any given movement. These are just a few examples but the possibilities to craft a solid strength training program are endless.

I don't recommend 1RM test for beginners for at least 6 months after they've begun consistent weight training. You can go heavy, but your focus should be on form and technique. You'll run the risk of injury because your brain's ability to control the lift while maintaining proper midline stabilization will not be developed yet. Be patient and remember this isn't a "6 weeks to a six pack" kind of thing. This is a lifelong practice and if you're serious then you need to allow time for your training to mature.

HIIT vs. Endurance

"Blur the distinction between strength training and metabolic conditioning for the simple reason that nature's challenges are typically blind to the distinction."

-Coach Glassman founder of CrossFit

For many years the general consensus on improving one's cardiovascular health was to simply increase the volume of endurance exercise such as running or cycling. The thinking was that some is good, but more is better. Marathon runners and long distance cyclist graced the cover of fitness magazines, being touted as the fittest people on earth. While very impressive, research is finding that the benefits we seek from an improved cardiovascular system (such as lower resting heart rate, lower body fat, greater endurance, better sleep and overall improved health) can be accessed much more rapidly with High Intensity Interval Training (HIIT), and with less of the downside often associated with chronic endurance training.

In a 2008 training study by Burgomaster et al at the National Center for Biotechnology Information, subjects were divided into two groups of 5 men and 5 women per group. For 6 weeks one group performed 4-6 repeats of 30 second all out sprints on a stationary bike followed by 4.5 minutes of rest 3 times per week.

The next group performed 40-60 minutes of cycling at 65% of their VO2 max, 5 days per week. At the end of the study both groups experienced similar metabolic adaptations responsible for effective breakdown of carbohydrates and fats along with an improved VO2 max. The striking difference between these two groups was the amount of time actually spent training. The 40-60 minute endurance group spent approximately 4.5 hours per week cycling in order to see the same results the sprinting group achieved with only 1.5 hours per week of cycling.

Using the same model, you could replace cycling with any movement and achieve greater metabolic adaptations than with endurance training alone.

The potential downside of chronic endurance training, especially long distance running, is the wear and tear on joints along with prolonged levels of metabolic stress. High cortisol levels are found in endurance athletes which leads to the breakdown of muscle tissue as the body converts it into glycogen for fuel. This usually leads to the spare tire around many endurance athlete's midsection and has baffled those who think that running 50 miles a week will turn them into a lean machine. In fact, research is finding more and more evidence to the contrary, pointing to short, intense bouts of HIIT as the optimal prescription for healthy biomarkers and metabolic adaptations.

Long distance running tends to be hard on the body. Not necessarily because of the modality itself, but due to the breakdown of proper form many experience as the muscle tissues fatigue. This breakdown isn't exclusive to running and can be seen with any type of continuous exertion lasting longer than 20 minutes.

Running a couple of miles at a time for proficiency or heading out to the track for some sprint repeats is an entirely different physiological animal than a 60-minute slug. I understand that this may not be welcomed news for some of you out there who live for insane feats of endurance, but I'm not saying we shouldn't do it whatsoever. Just pointing back to the research done around equivalent metabolic adaptations with literally a fourth of the amount of time spent training. Less time spent equals less wear and tear, and more time for training other beneficial aspects of fitness.

A long run or ride every so often is totally fine and serves as a welcomed break from the gym. It's only a problem when it becomes the default mode of training. In my 13 years of coaching the two types of people I see with the greatest physical dysfunctions are those who chronically run and/or cycle and, and those who sit at a desk all day.

At this point we understand that the body is incredibly adaptive for better or for worse. In essence, it's why we build muscle, lose fat, lose muscle and build fat. When we introduce a stimulus or lack thereof, our body goes to work adapting to it by becoming stronger, leaner or fatter.

However, if we do not vary the stimulus we will fall victim to the law of accommodation (discussed earlier in this chapter) which states that if the external stimulus does not vary our body will accommodate and decrease in strength and ability.

Endurance based training especially tends to become stale rather quickly due to the relatively low levels of intensity and the lack of variation required to sustain it. By the very nature of the oxidative pathway responsible for fueling this type of activity, intensity levels never reach more than 75% of maximal heart rate; because there's no real shock to the system, the body adapts very quickly to the stimulus which leads to diminishing returns.

Whereas the first dozen or so runs may leave you totally wiped out and sore for days, within a relatively short period the same old 10k will cease to have the effect on you it once did. Whatever results you may have seen in the beginning will likely undo themselves as your body acclimates to its new normal. Don't get me wrong here. Proficiency in all areas of exercise is the goal, but the low intensity, repetitiveness nature of endurance training actually harms your potential as an athlete much the same way packing on too much unnecessary muscles without correlating strength ratios will.

Using high intensity interval training, on the other hand, gives you the ability to improve your metabolic condition to the levels of top endurance athletes in a fraction of the time. It also allows for the incorporation of an ever changing variety of movements, time modalities, loads and distances to ensure muscle confusion and the subsequent adaptation responses.

Basically, your options are endless with HIIT (high intensity interval training). You're only limited by your own creativity. Within a single 60 minute training session you can reap the benefits of a full strength and conditioning workout without having to designate entire sessions for one or the other. In other words, intensity is way more effective than volume; it also tends to be the holy grail for results. Nothing gets the hormones pumping like and all out sprint and that's exactly what is needed for our body to mobilize those stubborn fat deposits and start channeling the calories we consume into new muscle tissue.

In the study above a stationary bike may have been used to complete interval sprints but do not thing that you are you limited to cycling. High intensity interval training can be described as a period of high intensity followed by a period of low to moderate intensity, for instance, 20 burpees as fast as possible followed by a 400-meter run for 4 rounds, or 10 heavy deadlifts and15 pull-ups followed by 100 skips on the jump rope for 5 rounds. These are classic examples of HIIT because they are short, intense and highly effective at increasing one's athleticism as well as improving one's metabolism.

How to run

After reading the last section you might think I am against running, but I'm not. In fact, I really enjoy it. Nothing gets me ready for a hard workout like running a mile first. Although I prefer shorter sprints to long distance, I do see value in the occasional run over 20 minutes.

So, if we're going to do it we might as well do it right, right?

Step 1: Get Off Your Heels

Do you or someone you know get shin splints when they run? If you take a look at a foot, you'll notice a couple of things. One, is that the heel resembles a blunt force object that offers little to no shock absorption ability. Though this may be great for side kicking an intruder in the gut or breaking a 2x4 it is not so great for absorbing the impact of your bodyweight repeatedly while running.

The toes on the other hand are a web of joints, tendons, ligaments and muscle perfectly designed to disperse the weight of your body as you strike the ground. The arch of your foot acts as a spring shooting you forward with every stride. In addition to the arch of your foot acting as a spring when you practice a forefoot strike, the achilles tendon acts as a second spring propelling you forward.

However, if your first point of contact with the ground while running is with your heel, then you're essentially stunting the reactive - plyometric force that generates as the toes, arch and achilles engage to spring us forward with maximum efficiency. Heel striking slows down your run speed, creating more work for yourself. In a forefoot strike you reduce the amount of time your foot makes contact with the ground which translates to a faster, lighter stride.

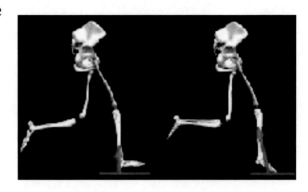

People often suffer from shin splints when the heel hits the ground like a baseball bat sending a shock wave up the lower leg. This inflames the tissues surrounding the tibia.

However, a forefoot (toe) strike shifts the runners center of mass forward allowing them to keep their joints stacked and proper muscles engaged. The heel strike on the other hand shifts your center of mass behind your stride so you're reaching your leg forward to the ground with every stride instead of being over your hips and striking the ground beneath you.

I know some people will argue this point, but a quick way to demonstrate that heel running is inferior, and only exists because of the cushion on the heel of nearly all running shoes, is to have someone run barefoot. They might make it an 8th of a mile before they'll have to shift to their toes or stop all together.

Basically nobody heel strikes barefoot. Up until recently it wasn't uncommon to find many track programs teaching a heel strike due to the lack of research done on this topic. However, after an increase medical and sports experts began testing this theory the consensus has changed; now a forefoot strike is often taught and practiced by track athletes.

The graph below highlight the power lost from heel striking

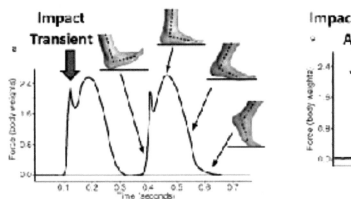

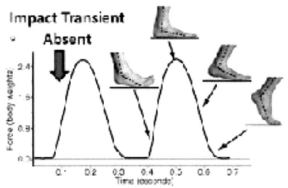

Less is more

Thanks to books like, "Born to Run" By Chris McDougall the mainstream view has changed rapidly. In his book, McDougall detailed the reasons heel striking is a symptom of a larger problem: the running shoe industry. He explains how in the 1970s Nike literally invented the running shoe and adorned it with an inch of foam padding under the heel that not only enabled people to begin heel striking but raised the heel higher than the toe, creating an unnatural heel-toe differential. Having a wedge under the heel shifts your center of mass forward in passive body positions like standing or walking, thus creating a front/back asymmetry by overloading the quadriceps and inhibiting the glutes.

McDougall points out that the thick cushioning also dulls the tactile sensors in the feet which relay information to the brain about the firmness and texture of the ground your walking or running on. He points out that the feet actually have more of these sensors than the hands and face, and dictate how hard we strike the ground.

Using pressure sensing treadmills researchers found that due to the extra thick padding on most running shoes, participants struck the treadmill much harder causing greater shockwaves up the leg. Those wearing firmer or minimal footwear ran more gracefully and experienced less impact.

This seems counter intuitive but the brain is always aiming to find balance and if the signals from your feet are dulled due to the softness of your shoe, then your brain will want you to slam that foot down harder so it can get a read of the surface that you're on.

I recommend forefoot running with minimal padding to my clients. For those who are accustomed to the old school extra thick, heel strike promoting running shoe, the transition to a flat harder shoe can be tough. Your legs will most likely ache from the change in tension dispersion. However, if you can keep yourself strong during the acclimation phase you will save yourself from a lot of trouble down the road. No pun intended.

Over Training

This is a touchy subject. Diehards hate when people suggest that they might be over training or that the results they're getting could be achieved with less work and a sharper focus on nutrition.

They might brush it off and say something like, "You just don't understand." Or, "I enjoy training like this." Fair enough, but my goal with this book is to show you a path towards fitness without having to kill yourself in the process. I want a sustainable approach that will keep me lean and strong for the rest of my life without the physical and mental stress of practically having a second job of training myself in the gym. This is possible.

Throughout my life I've had the opportunity to argue both sides of this debate. When I used to train for kickboxing competitions it was 3 hours a day, 5 days a week. Yes, I was fast, powerful, and totally ripped but I was also totally exhausted. As an athlete, my general well-being had become second to my performance.

It didn't matter that I was a moody dick who needed 20 minutes in the morning before I could stand up straight due to a tight back and hips, as long as I could go into the ring and kick ass. Regardless, you better believe I would have debated you all day on the importance of my training volume, and due to the demands of the sport there was merit to it. However, now that I am the one coaching younger athletes, I see the same patterns unfolding that I experienced in kickboxing: being averse to taking a day off for fear of the competition getting an edge on you.

Social media pages filled with dogmatic passages like "train the pain away" and "pain is just weakness leaving your body" don't help the issue. Catchy sure, but you have to ask yourself how much is enough, and where exactly is the point of diminishing returns?

The vast majority of us are over training because we believe this is how you get healthy, strong and look great, not necessarily because we have any athletic ambitions.

In other words, a professional athlete will train 3-5 hours a day not because she seeks to be more "fit", but because she needs to gain mastery of a skill set with improved accuracy, balance and whatever specific technique the sport requires. Being an athlete is her job and she must treat it as such.

For the rest of us with families, careers and deadlines, without the proper support system a training regimen like this can leave our bodies exhausted and achy. You may start to look good and experience results, but what good are those results if the volume of work it takes to get them is unsustainable? One of the saddest things is someone stuck in perpetual yo-yoing because of the unrealistic expectations they've placed on themselves.

It's tough not to buy into the idea that more is better. The internet abounds with movie stars that got totally ripped for a movie role, and when you hear about their story its almost always a tale of extreme dieting and spending 2 hours a day in the gym. The fact is that if you only have a few months to completely change your body then extreme times call for extreme measures. The ability to get completely shredded in a short period of time absolutely exist. Those actors had a team of trainers and nutritionists working with them daily in order to prepare for the big shirtless scene.

Within weeks of the movie wrapping, however, those results begin to fade away if the volume is not kept up, some faster than others depending on their genetics. The shear amount of work and precision required for those extreme transformations are next to impossible to maintain for a long period of time.

Don't be discouraged though. You can get amazing results that last without having to go to extremes. As with so many things in life, consistency is the key. When creating the perfect program, it's important to ask yourself what is the minimum effective dose?

You'd be hard pressed to find many sports science academics who argue that more is *always* better. My personal opinion is that we should push the envelope without ripping it. Let your capacity to train harder increase naturally. If you're new to exercise, the foundation you build your practice on should be intended to last a lifetime. Rushing it and pushing yourself to the extreme is a sure way to burnout before you get to where you want to be.

Training volumes should change to facilitate the greatest adaptational response. For example, after a few hard weeks of exercise, a lighter "de-load" week can be incredibly beneficial. If a routine is becoming stale then yes, a few super intense workouts might be just the thing to get you back on track. Conversely, if you're feeling burned out then a few days off might be exactly what you need to feel great again. The bottom line is that there is no one way about it. We just need to make sure we look forward to our time in the gym and not grow to resent it.

If you're feeling stressed, achy, weak, moody, chronically fatigued, dehydrated, always on the brink of a cold, susceptible to infections and experiencing headaches or tremors these could all be signs of overtraining. Overtraining creates an addictive relationship towards exercise, and alters the function of the immune system and central nervous system. Elevated cortisol levels, due to over training, leads to metabolism dysfunction. Micro-trauma to the muscles can also occur faster than the body can repair them. Although true "Over Training Syndrome" (OTS) is rare, it can happen and you should know what signs to look for just in case. The best cure is hydration, nutrition, massage and most importantly, rest.

Hormones

In this book, I've previously referred to various hormones. Since you can't really talk about training without talking about our hormonal system it's time to dive into this topic with a little more detail.

It's important to understand how much our hormones impact our body composition (the ratio between fat and muscle), mood, strength, sleep and fertility. Hormones come and go, raise and lower daily based on how we sleep, what we eat and drink, how much or how little exercise we get, how much sex we have, how old we are, how we deal with stress, how we feel about ourselves, and even how we come across to others.

The hormones that promote muscle growth and fat loss are testosterone, IGF-1, growth hormone and insulin. On the other hand, cortisol and glucagon promote muscle breakdown. Cortisol also contributes to fat storage. The main hormones responsible for fat loss are growth hormone, glucagon, testosterone, noradrenaline and adrenaline.

While there is way more to hormones than we will be able to cover here, lets break down some of the more popular ones to see what their jobs are and how to control them.

Growth Hormone (GH)

GH is a highly behavioral hormone and is release when we experience low blood sugar. Low blood sugar results from exercise, fasting, dieting and sleep. When produced, this hormone helps build and maintain muscle through protein synthesis and by mobilizing fat that had been stored to use as fuel.

Therefore, higher GH levels protect against muscle loss. The presence of GH lowers the amount of glucose and protein your body uses for fuel by burning up fat instead.

IGF-1 (another important anabolic hormone) is released alongside of GH. Production of this hormone by the anterior pituitary gland peaks around age 20 with your body releasing around 500 micrograms a day, and declines rapidly after age 30 by about 24% per decade. You can help keep GH production high by getting a good 7-9 hours of sleep a night, keeping your workouts short and intense, and keeping your blood sugars low.

Testosterone

Although women's adrenal glands produce a small amount of this hormone, testosterone, produced by male testes, is the predominant hormone for muscle growth in men. It also helps define sexual characteristics and burns fat.

Per a study in The Journal of Applied Physiology called "Influences of Testosterone On Muscle Mass and Protein Synthesis":

> "Testosterone directly stimulates protein synthesis resulting in muscle growth. Around age 40 tends to be when men experience large declines in testosterone production under normal circumstances resulting in higher body fat and lower muscle and bone density."

All is not lost though! Low carb/high fat diets and weight training promote higher than average levels of testosterone. Cholesterol in food is directly responsible for the production of testosterone. Much like GH, we can naturally increase our levels by getting good sleep, keeping a cool-calm-collected demeanor, eating a high protein/fat/low carb diet, and hitting the weights.

Insulin

Insulin is a storage hormone. Your body's two main storage depots happen to be muscle and fat, so depending on your eating and exercise habits insulin can work for or against you.

Insulin promotes muscle growth as well as fat storage. Its main job is to keep blood glucose levels down. When we eat carbs, fat or protein a portion of those calories are released into the blood stream as glucose. This rise in blood sugar (glucose) triggers the pancreas to release insulin so it can find a place to store those glucose molecules. Too much glucose in the blood is dangerous and could be lethal, which is why insulin is so important.

Insulin promotes muscle growth by blunting the breakdown of muscle tissue into fuel. It forces glucose into the muscle tissue, which stimulates protein synthesis. Conversely, consistently high glucose levels directly correlate with body fat storage, and consistently low insulin levels can hinder muscle growth to a degree.

Because of this, the only way to truly control your body fat and muscle mass is to control your insulin levels. The best way to control your insulin levels is by controlling your diet.

Although all food converts into glucose to some degree and causes a rise in insulin, **carbohydrates** have the largest effect on insulin levels because the body converts them directly into blood sugar, especially when eaten alone.

When eaten alone, the liver converts only a little over 50% of the **proteins** we eat are converted into blood glucose. However, the percentage lowers when eaten with carbohydrates because the body prefers carbs for this purpose. **Fat** has an even lower blood glucose conversion rate at around 10%, which is hardly enough to matter.

This is why a high carb/protein post workout shake is often recommended. Since your muscle's glycogen stores are depleted post workout, you can take full advantage of insulin's anabolic power by channeling proteins and sugars to your muscles without the excess glucose calories spilling over into body fat. All other times blood glucose levels should remain low.

IGF-1

Insulin- like growth factor 1 (IGF-1) has an anabolic effect on nearly every cell in the body: skeletal muscles, bone, cartilage, liver, skin, kidneys, nerves and lungs.

This hormone peaks around puberty and is a key factor for tissue growth. According to a study done by Molecular Endocrinology Volume 6, Number 11 entitled, "Growth Hormone Rapidly Activates Insulin Like Growth Factor 1 Gene transcription in Vivo", the release of IGF-1, which is produced by the liver, is triggered when growth hormone is high. Here's the tricky part though: Because IGF-1 is similar to insulin in form and function AND works in tandem with growth hormone, it is released by the liver during times of elevated levels of GH AND insulin.

Since we know that GH production is blunted by high levels of insulin but IGF-1 is not released without the presents of insulin, the best way to capitalize on this powerful anabolic hormone is with a high carb/protein shake immediately following an intense workout.

For example, post workout your GH levels are through the roof so by downing a high carb/protein shake within 30 minutes of completing your workout you'll trigger the release of insulin, which in turn triggers the release of IGF-1.

Cortisol

Unlike IGF-1, insulin, testosterone, and growth hormone (which are all considered anabolic hormones that promote tissue growth), cortisol is a catabolic hormone often called the "stress hormone".

This hormone is released by the adrenal cortex during periods of physical and mental stress and plays a large part in the breakdown of muscle and the accumulation of body fat. Cortisol is the "fight or flight" hormone. In times of great stress the release of cortisol shuts down our metabolism, rapidly breaks down muscle tissue and converts it into glucose. That glucose supplies the brain with immediate fuel to quickly think our way out of a sticky situation, an incredibly valuable evolutionary process in acute moments of stress

However, chronically elevated levels of cortisol from prolonged mental and physical stress is incredibly damaging to our DNA. Inadequate sleep, high carbohydrate diets, work or family stress, and training sessions lasting over an hour raise cortisol production to unhealthy levels. This behavior also inhibits the production of beneficial hormones like GH and testosterone. Good sleep, healthy diets, short intense workouts and stress management are sure fire ways to keep cortisol levels in check.

Glucagon

Glucagon has an inverse relationship with insulin, when one is up the other is down. Whereas insulin takes glucose out of the blood and into muscles, liver and fat stores, glucagon takes glycogen out of the liver and mobilizes fat stores for energy.

Whereas insulin's job is to ensure blood sugar levels don't get too high, glucagon's job is to make sure blood sugar levels don't get too low. In some cases, it might convert amino acids from our muscle tissues into glucose if need be.

This hormone is important for those seeking to lose body fat through low carb diets because of its role in the breakdown of body fat for fuel. However, this also correlates with the breakdown in muscle tissue, and is why when you engage in a fat loss program you often lose a little muscle as well. Conversely, when you engage in a muscle building program you often add a little body fat.

The actual ratios of body fat and muscle mass accumulation or breakdown when engaging in either program depends greatly on meal timing, training intensity and your particular set of genes.

Adrenaline and Noradrenalin

(also referred to as epinephrine and norepinephrine)

Like cortisol these hormones are produced by the adrenal glands and are released during times of stress. As part of the "fight or flight" system, these hormones are responsible for increasing blood flow to muscles, heart rate, blood sugar and dilation of the pupils.

Subjects in a 1987 study done by the Journal of Clinical Investigation titled "Lipolysis During Fasting Decreased Suppression by Insulin and Increased Stimulation by Epinephrine", subjects experienced increased blood flow and breakdown of body fat when the cell receptors for these hormones were stimulated and insulin levels were low.

These hormones play a huge role is how much body fat one loses, and are triggered during exercise. Noradrenaline levels remain especially high long after your workout and explains how we continue to burn calories long after we finish training.

T3 & T4

Produced by the thyroid gland, these hormones regulate the metabolism of every cell in the body. Although the thyroid produces about 4 times more T4 than T3, T3 is about 4 times stronger. T3 has the greatest influence over your metabolism. High T3 levels increase your metabolism which can lead to both lower body fat levels as well as difficulty trying to gain muscle mass for hard gainers.

The amount of food you eat plays a large role in how much T3 your thyroid produces. Low calorie diets can reduce T3 levels by as much as 30%, lowering your metabolism to promote energy conservation when calories are at a deficit.

This explains how some overweight people struggle to lose weight even with a reduced calorie diet. Eating a consistently high caloric diet raises T3 levels which in turn increases your metabolism. This back and forth of rising and lowering of T3 levels is evolution's way of maintaining our body weight during times of feast or famine.

Low T3 means a very slow metabolism which means no fat is being burned. Since T3 also aids in protein synthesis; low levels stall any new muscle growth. So keep this hormone up by consistent exercise and a healthy diet of cycling carbs on and off, depending on your activity levels. Refer back to the chapter on nutrition for a more in-depth look at carb cycling.

These are just a few of the many hormones that control the functions of our body. To address them all or even half would be an entire book of its own. However, from this list we can at least see how our behavior inhibits or elicits the hormones that help govern our metabolism. Hormones have the power to change the way we think, feel, look and desire. Understanding them on a deeper level will guide our decision making when it comes to what we eat and how we spend our time in the gym.

Sample Month Of Training

Performance Code - Month 1

Weeks 1-3
Increase weight 3-5% weekly

Monday

a) Front Squats: 5 sets of 5 reps every 2 1/2 minutes

b) Back squats: 1 set of 12 reps @ 80% of front squat weight

c) Strict Barbell Shoulder Press: 8 sets of 3 reps every 2 minutes

d) 5 minute EMOM (every minute on the minute): 10 dumbbell push presses.

e) 8 minute AMRAP (as many rounds as possible): 10 dumbbell snatches, 10 pushups, 15 v-ups.

Wednesday

a) Deadlifts: 5 sets of 3 reps every 2 1/2 minutes

b) Max effort weighted pull ups: 4 sets - pick a weight.

c) Kipping pull-ups: 20 reps

d) Bent over row: 4 sets of 5 reps

e) 8 minute EMOM: 1) 10 bicep curls 2) 10 dips

f) 9 minute AMRAP: 5 burpees, 10 24" box jumps, 20 sit ups

Friday:

a) Back Rack Lunges 5 sets of 10 reps every 2 minutes.

b) Flat barbell bench press: 10-8-6-4-2-12

c) Seated dumbbell Press: 5x5

d) 10 minute EMOM: 1) 10 lateral raises 2) 10 skull crushers

e) 10 minute AMRAP: 200m run, 15 KB swings, 10 toe to bar.

Saturday:

Interval sprints - Chose a new one every week.

30 seconds of all out effort every 2 minutes for 10 rounds of:

Running, cycling, punching the heavy bag, double unders, rowing or battle ropes.

Week 4 - De-load week

Monday

21-15-9 squat cleans, ring dips

Wednesday

21-15-9 Deadlifts, Hand stand push ups (shoulder press if you can't do hand stand push ups yet

Friday

20 minute AMRAP 5 pull-ups, 10 pushups, 15 squats.

Saturday

One mile run for time

Chapter 5

Movement Mechanics

"Poor movement can exist anywhere in the body, but poor movement patterns can only exist in the brain"

- Dr. Gray Cook. Founder of the Functional Movement Screen.

We're going to close out this book with a section on movement and mobility. Google defines mobility as, "The ability to move or be moved freely and easily." Being mobile doesn't just mean flexible. It implies a certain level of body control through range of motion in all joints.

I see a lot of people spend a ton of time stretching their hamstrings to the point where touching their toes is no problem. Yet, those same people still round their backs every time they bend over to pick something up from the ground. Simply "stretching out" doesn't equal good movement patterns. On the other hand, I've met people with terrible range of motion, yet move incredibly well. The difference is how well you not only understand proper movement mechanics, but practice them. Much like exercise, mobility is a practice. The only way to correct poor movement is to be aware of and actively participate with your body's positioning. All day, every day.

The ultimate expression of form and function is achieved when lengthening the muscle tissue through stretching and massage is combined with an awareness and practice of proper movement patterns.

Don't get me wrong here, stretching by itself isn't bad necessarily. However, you can be flexible as hell and still move like shit. As Grey Cook says, "You have to hit save on the document", meaning you have to understand proper movement patterns and hold yourself to a high standard of excellence in practicing them. Only then will lengthening the muscle have its greatest effect on your movement mechanics.

For example, in the pictures below you will see me in a deadlift sequence from beginning to end. With a braced core, I bend over to pick up the barbell. Hinging at the waist while maintaining a neutral spine, I keep the weight of my body in my heels with my shoulders in front of the bar and arms straight.

Focusing on these key points of performance in this lift makes you far less likely to suffer from back problems thanks to an understanding of proper movement mechanics and patterns. Increased flexibility in my hips is icing on the cake, but the real focus should be placed on developing better movement patterns.

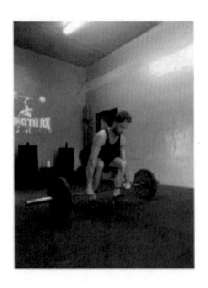 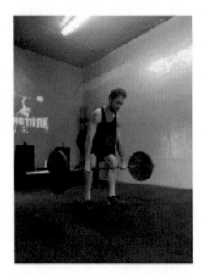 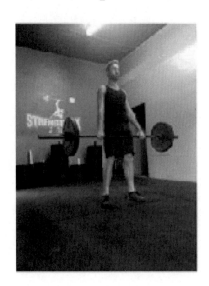

Midline Stabilization

"We should always be working towards achieving midline stabilization when training by neutralizing our entire spine from head to hips."

- Justin Schollard, The Performance Code

You hear many people say that the inability to maintain proper midline stabilization when training stems from one or both of the following: lack of hip strength and mobility and/or lack of shoulder strength and mobility. While these conditions can certainly hinder one's progress, it is my belief that a lack of understanding is at the heart of the issue. I have personally witnessed people with awful range of motion and muscular development hit a perfect squat, deadlift and overhead press with the right cuing.

It is our current state of evolution that is to blame for this lack of movement proficiency. As technology advances and makes our lives more and more convenient, we now have to deliberately train the very movement patterns that separated us from the rest of the animal kingdom.

Because of this, it is now our obligation to make a concerted effort towards maintaining midline stability and proper form whether we're exercising or simply picking a bag up from the floor. Without this practice our body will always divert tension away from the less developed patterns and into the more developed ones.

For example, if every time you deadlift your head snaps back, back rounds or knees buckle then you are essentially training yourself to lift this way, and will always default to this movement pattern at the slightest sign of fatigue.

This is what Dr. Grey Cook, founder of the Functional Movement Screen (FMS), calls "high tension strategies". In other words, it's the way your body finds joint stability for better or for worse. Unfortunately, our body doesn't think about the long term safety of movement patterns. It doesn't say to it's self, "I should really stop snapping my head back when I deadlift, allowing my knees to buckle in when I squat or letting my hips sag when I do push-ups because in ten years this might turn into a problem."

On the contrary, If we do not intervene and correct the course of our movement pattern development then our survival instincts will govern our mechanics, especially in high stress situations.

For example, when you're grinding through a heavy squat and the alarm bells are ringing in your head, what's the fasted way to get a quick 2 inches out of the bottom? Buckle your knees. Any one time and you'll likely come out just fine. However, when allowed to happen repeatedly a very fast recruitment order establishes itself between squatting and buckling knees. This then becomes your default movement pattern because whether you know it or not you've trained yourself this way. If left unchecked this could lead to serious knee problems which feeds the fire around whether squatting is good for you or not.

Again, the movements themselves aren't bad, but the way they are done absolutely could be. This is why real strength training is a skill. As conscious beings we must be in control of our physical positions at all times.

The Bracing Sequence

Hands down the best preventative measure for this is what Dr. Kelly Starrett coined as the "bracing sequence".

Before every lift run through this check list and you'll be in the top ten percent of people who lift with best practices; fill your lungs with air, squeeze your butt muscles, squeeze your abs and tuck your chin. Now you're braced and in the best possible position to perform any lift.

The bracing sequence locks in your core in place by stabilizing your pelvis in a neutral position. This neutral pelvic position combined with tight abs ensures that the lumbar spine is protected and neutral as the hips do their job of flexing and extending.

When this is not practiced the pelvis is loose and abs are soft, the lumbar spine takes the brunt of the load. This has the potential to cause a slew of issues including tweaked low back muscles due to overcompensation from inactive glutes, herniated disks, or vertebrae damage. This can also lead to bone spurs due to repeated overarching under load of the lumber spine.

Don't let this scare you. Simply by taking a little time each day to mobilize your joints and practicing the bracing sequence along with proper movement mechanics you will reprogram your mind and body to recruit the right muscles every time. Before long it will become second nature…again.

Fitness Doesn't Grant You Immunity

"Don't layer fitness over dysfunction" - Gray Cook.

We had a young guy join our gym a couple years back who showed the greatest promise of all the aspiring athletes we've had walk through our door. He was 25, an ex-football player, college wrestler and had specific coaching in olympic lifting.

He walked in deadlifting over 500 pounds, squatting over 400 pounds and benching in the high 300s. He was a beast and we were stoked to have him. Other members stared in awe at his feats of strength and there became a feeling in the gym that he could do no wrong.

The coaching staff even bought into it for a while. However, as the weeks went on we started noticing small faults in his lifting, and it soon became clear that if his habits continued, unchecked, it would become a real problem. One day he revealed to us that he in fact deals with constant low back pain. At the point when his strength levels were through the roof, we knew we had to pull him back from the volume he was training at before it was too late.

Thankfully, he was a good sport and respected our advice to take a step back in order to examine his lifts and clear up his movement patterns. We discovered that he had a bad habit of overarching his spine whenever he back squatted or snatched. In his defense, this is totally common, and to his credit he took perfecting his midline stabilization very seriously.

This was a guy who could back squat 400 pounds cold and was now using the empty bar, drilling the movement with zero flux in his spine. It was awesome to watch. He took a big step back to correct his movements and is now squatting, deadlifting, and snatching the same if not more than he was 6 months ago. The only difference is this time he's doing it with great form.

Lo and behold, back pain is gone. It's hard to put a halt to your momentum when your strength levels are going up, even if you're in pain. You must abandon your ego and go back to basics, but it's the only way to truly reprogram how your body recruits muscle groups.

Because he took action and cleaned up his movements he has enabled himself to become an even better athlete. Dr. Kelley Starrett estimates that if your mobility is poor then you're working about ten percent harder to get your joints in the correct position than if you were mobile and could move freely through range of motion. Ten percent could mean the difference between winning or losing. This is why we say, "Stiffness is weakness." Gray Cook says it best: "Sometimes it's easier to take the hand break off than to keep hitting the gas pedal."

Myofascial Pain (trigger points) Causes and Solutions

I am not a doctor. Please do not consider this to be a diagnosis of any kind but simply a list of mobility practices that I have compiled through years of trial, error, independent study and pattern recognition.

These methods are to treat trigger points which occur in the belly (thickest part) of the muscle and are usually a result of stiffness, overuse and poor posture. Trigger points refer pain to other areas of the body that can feel extremely painful and make it tricky to identify where they originate.

More commonly referred to as "muscle knots", trigger points develop when a patch of muscles fibers is in spasm [Wikipedia]. When you get a trigger point developing in an area its usually a sign that blood flow and mobility are hindered. A power loss will likely follow and irritation of the surrounding areas will occur if not corrected. This could also lead to compensation and poor movement patterns as your body protects the injured area. Because of the severity of the pain, people often mistake trigger points for torn muscles, nerve damage or joint damage.

If trigger points get bad enough it can turn into Myofascial Pain Syndrome (MPS) which is defined as several bundles of muscles fibers in spasm. MPS and Fibromyalgia are almost identical in symptoms and for that reason hard to tell apart.

There is no quick fix, only sound practices and principals. Even the best therapist cannot fix you in one or two sessions. It's through dedicated self-effort that one begins to fully understand how their body works and how to optimize it. Let's take a look at a few common areas of the body where trigger points develop and some techniques for mobilization and pain relief.

It should be noted that the sum is greater than its parts, and although some muscles groups and joints effect each other more directly, an imbalance in one has a chain reaction throughout your entire body.

Stiff shoulders will cause compensation from your lower back, stiff hips will make it difficult to keep your shoulders from rolling forward, so on and so forth. We have to look at our body holistically and understand that everything effects everything. Nothing is isolated in nature and that includes how our body moves.

Shoulders, Upper Back and Neck

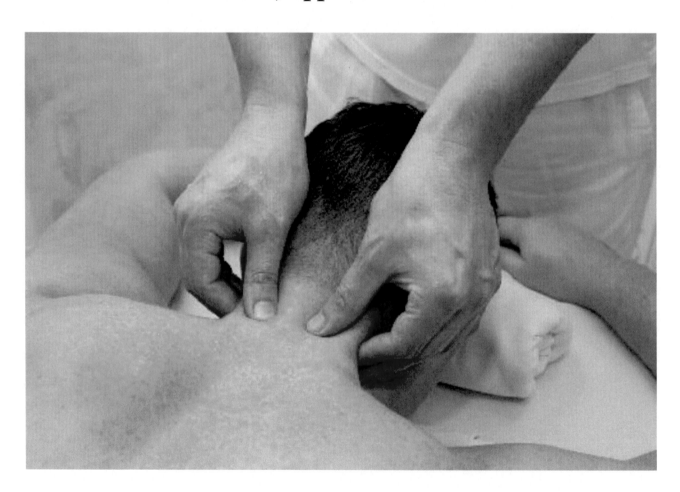

I hear the most complaints of pain originating around this area. The neck, shoulders and upper back are so intimately related that you can't really talk about one without mentioning the other.

Although there is no definitive study, researchers are linking migraines and other forms of headaches with myofascial problems in the neck and shoulders. Rounded shoulders and a forward protruding head is probably one of the most common problems I see.

When the shoulders are rounded it exacerbates the muscles of the upper back and shoulders (traps, rear delts, rhomboids, rotators, lavator and erectors) by keeping them in a constant loaded position. Over time this position weakens and pain can develop in the form of trigger points.

On the other side of your body, the pectoral muscles of the chest shorten as the shoulders gradually roll further and further forward, creating a vicious cycle of weak posterior muscles of the upper back and stiff short pectoral muscles of the chest. This significantly reduces your shoulder's range of motion, forcing your body to overextend at the lumbar spine whenever you try to extend your arms over your head.

Below is a simple 3 step process to mobilize your shoulders, upper back and neck.

Step 1:
Massage Your Pectoral Muscles

In this picture you see a lacrosse ball wedged between my upper peck muscles and the wall. After 2-3 minutes of firm intentional massage on each side I will move onto:

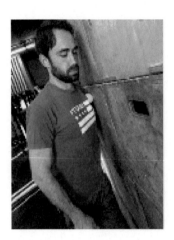 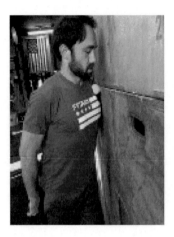

Step 2: Foam Roll Your Lats

After my painful pec massage I will now move on to foam rolling my lats. Just like pecs, the lats can be a huge inhibitor of full shoulder range of motion. Spend about 2-3 minutes rolling out each side, then move onto picture 3.

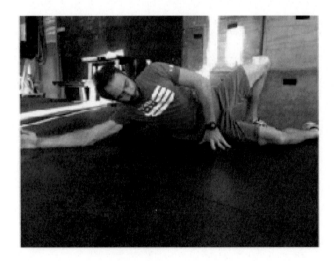 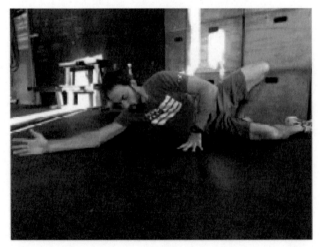

Step 3: Stretch Your Pecs

Once my pecs and lats are sufficiently massaged and foam rolled, it's time to stretch them. On a flat bench with 3-5 pound dumbbells in my hands I straighten my arms out over my chest and lower them down, as if doing a fly, until I reach my end range of motion. Here, I will breath calmly and deeply, allowing the weight of the dumbbells to pull my arms closer to the floor and settling into a deep chest stretch. Hold this stretch for about a minute.

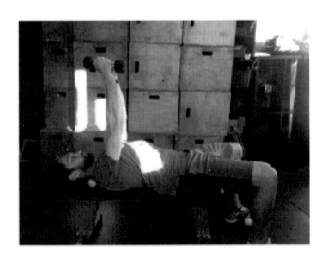 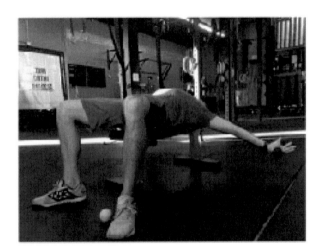

If you find yourself with stiff/achy shoulders, follow this simple protocol 3-4 times per week. Remember though, all the foam rolling and stretching in the world won't fix your shoulders if proper posture and movement patterns are not practiced.

Hips and lower back

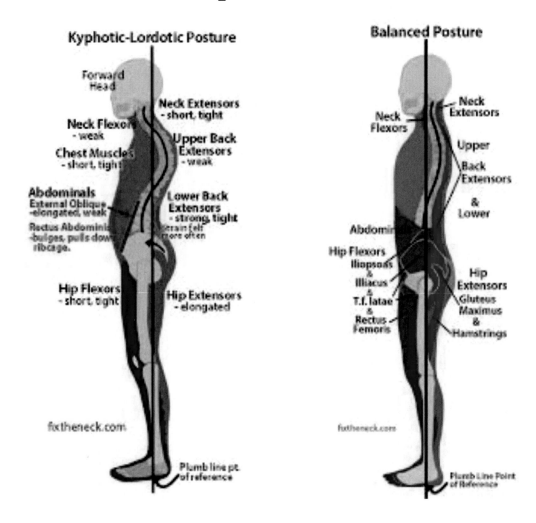

Rarely is back pain caused by the back itself. Pain in your back is a symptom of poor hip/shoulder mobility and movement patterns. If the muscles in your hip (mainly hamstrings, quadriceps, gluteus, adductor and flexors) are stiff or inhibited then your lower back is recruited by your brain to pick up the slack.

The number one cause of this is prolonged sitting. Dr. Peter T. Katzmarzyk led researchers on a study to determine the effects of prolonged sitting and sedentary behavior that was featured in the July 10th, 2012 issue of the Wall Street Journal. He estimates sitting for 3 hours or more a day can decrease your life expectancy by 2 years, even if you're physically active, eat well and do not smoke or drink.

By my estimations this is nearly the entire developed world (myself included). Siting is destructive for many reasons; it inhibits your glutes, which are the main muscles responsible for extending your hips when you run, walk, stand, lunge, jump, kick etc. When you sit on these poor guys all day your body, the clever creature it is, starts recruiting other muscles to do the job. Over time this leads to a cascade of postural issues and causes pain when you do just about anything but sit, so sitting becomes the dominate position your body feels best in, a self-perpetuating cycle of increased sitting and back pain.

Since we know that movement is the number one thing we can do to heal and rejuvenate our body, it would make sense then that the opposite is also true. A sedentary lifestyle will slowly kill us.

The best thing you can do for your hips and back is to be active, move every hour and follow the steps in this process to increase range of motion.

Step 1:

Massage Those Glutes!

In this step, take a lacrosse ball and lay over the top of it. With the ball between your butt and the floor, spend 3 minutes on each glute, slowly rolling all areas of the muscle.

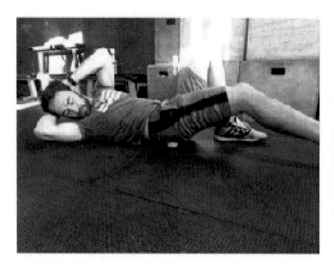 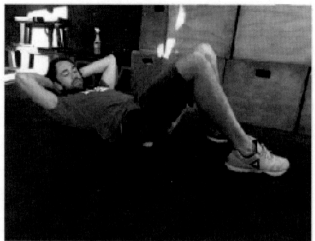

Step 2:

Stretch Those Gultes!

After you have sufficiently massaged each side with the ball, hold yourself in a pigeon stretch for 1 minute each side.

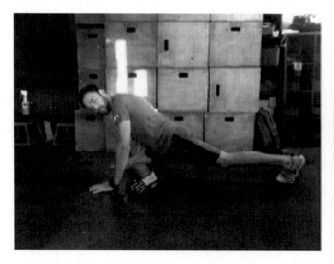 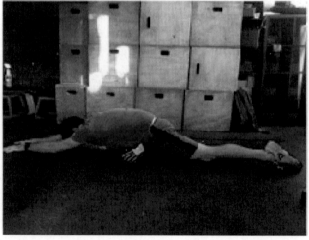

Step 3:
Roll Those Quads!

After your pigeon stretch it's time to go after the front side of your hips. Sitting, in addition to inhibiting your glute also shortens the muscles of the anterior (front) hip. For that reason, we will now foam roll each quadricep all the way up to the hip crease and all the way down to the knee. Repeat this slow deliberate rolling for 3 minutes each side.

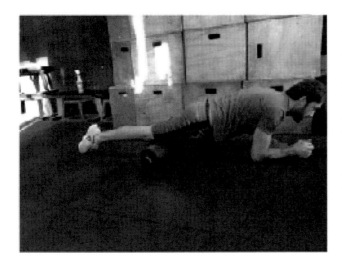 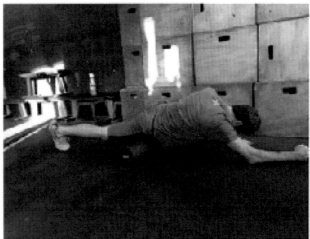

Step 4:
Stretch Those Quads!

After you've rolled the hell out of your quads it's time to stretch them. Back up to a wall and place your knee directly in the corner of the floor and the wall. Try and get your shin flush with the wall and take a big step all the way forward with the other foot. Flex the glute of whatever leg is being stretched. Hold this for one minute each side.

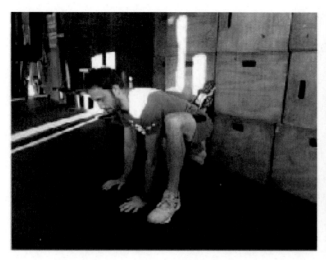 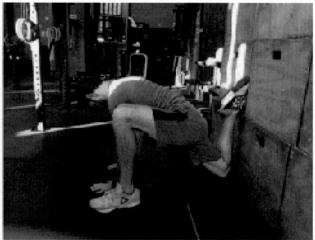

Step 5:

Bust Up Those Hammies!

Now that we have properly mobilized our glutes and quads it's time to dig into the hamstrings. Find a tall box or bench and place a lacrosse ball under your upper thigh just below your butt. From here you're going to apply downward pressure onto your hamstring and straighten out your knee. Move the ball one inch closer to your knee and repeat until you get to your knee and switch legs.

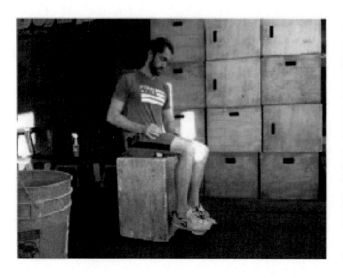 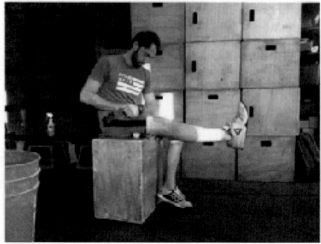

Step 6:
Stretch Those Hammies!

Last, but not least it's time to stretch our hamstrings. This one couldn't be more basic, but when done consistently is highly effective. Stand tall, reach your arms in the air, take a deep breath and bend over at the waist as you exhale and reach for your toes. Keep taking big breaths and reaching a little further with each exhale. Hold this for one minute.

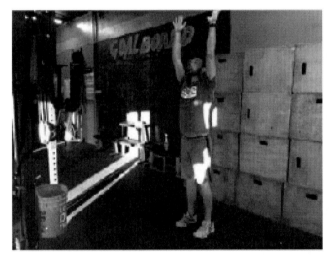 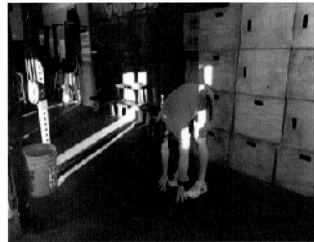

There is obviously way more to mobilizing your hips and shoulders than what I described here. However, this is a simple and effective starting point to increase range of motion in your primary joints, and to begin incorporating flexibility and proper movement patterns into your weekly routine.

Final Word

I have a personal client who is an accountant and let's just say he could stand to lose a few pounds. We are absolutely the odd couple. Not only in our appearance, but also in our upbringing and priorities. Despite all this we get along smashingly and engage in the most interesting conversations because the parallels be fitness and finance are staggering.

Here are two guys that took two different directions. My client, let's just call him Joe, has spent his entire life crunching numbers, pulling all nighters on complex corporate financials and completely disregarded his physical condition in the process.

Now, at age 44 he is firmly in the top 1% of income earners. Yet, wants nothing more than to be thin and feel confident in his body. He kicks himself for not giving a single thought to his health and fitness for the past 25 years and solely focusing on advancing his career. The "I'm too busy" excuse in full effect. No matter how much money Joe makes it's never enough. His priorities on career are too strong and his behaviors are so engrained that now, after years of training he still struggles with the routine and commitment it'd going to take for him to reach his goals.

Joe acts as if there is a scarcity of money and an abundance of time. Nothing could be further from the truth.

What advice does Joe give his young clients just starting their career? Save your money. Invest at least 10% so that you can have a secure future. Good advice. Something I adhere to as well.

Image what Joe would look like in 5 years if he invested 10% waking hours to his health. For 10 hours a week he planned his meals, exercised and stretched he would be a completely new man. Heck even if he invested 5% of his waking hours to his health and fitness he would be. I really hope for his sake he does because its never too late.

"The best time to plant an Oak Tree was 20 years ago. The second best time is now"

- Some Finance Guy

If you're one of the many who find themselves confused and overwhelmed with the deluge of information that surrounds the health fitness industry then this book is for you. Arm yourself with the knowledge and understanding of how to create a healthy, sustainable and effective fitness routine that will prepare you for life's challenges and unlock your genetic potential. **The Performance Code** is your roadmap to sound nutrition, functional strength, conditioning and mobilization. Inside these pages you'll discover the time tested wisdom and truth on how to build muscle, shred fat and feel absolutely great!

The Performance Code is the hybridization and inclusion of all sound movement practices arranged to best support you specific goals.

ABOUT THE AUTHOR:

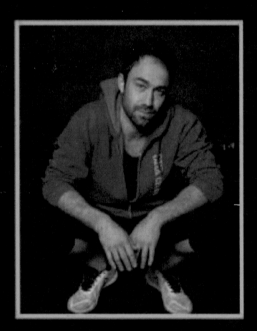

Justin Schollard has been a fitness coach and blogger in Los Angeles, CA for 13 years. He was the typical "skinny kid" growing up, but though years of dedicated work in both the gym and the kitchen he transformed himself into the athlete he knew he could be. Justin quickly became one of LA's top trainers and in 2013 opened his gym, StrengthRx, where he has literally helped thousands of budding athletes achieve their goals. In addition to the book, Justin also hosts The Performance Code podcast and online community where he shares his insights on health, fitness and lifestyle design to thousands on a weekly basis.

Check out www.PCodeNation.com and take the **FREE** course on how to increase your size, strength and athleticism.

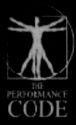

THE
PERFORMANCE
CODE

ID:223566
www.PCodeNation.com

87 869 5669 4663

Made in the USA
Middletown, DE
19 July 2017